ABC Relaxation Training

A Practical Guide for Health Professionals

Jonathan C. Smith, Ph.D.

 Springer Publishing Company
New York

Jonathan C. Smith, Ph.D., is a Licensed Clinical Psychologist, Distinguished Professor of Psychology, and founder and Director of the Roosevelt University Stress Institute. He has published numerous articles and 10 books on stress, relaxation, and meditation and has taught relaxation to thousands of individuals. Roosevelt University has granted Dr. Smith a Distinguished Professorship in order to conduct ABC relaxation research and develop the Stress Institute.

ABC Relaxation Training

A Practical Guide for Health Professionals

Jonathan C. Smith, Ph.D.

Springer Publishing Company, Inc.
536 Broadway
New York, NY 10012-3955

Acquisitions Editor: Bill Tucker
Production Editor: Helen Song
Cover design by James Scotto-Lavino

00 01 02 03 / 5 4 3 2

Library of Congress Cataloging-in-Publication Data

Smith, Jonathan C.
    ABC relaxation training : a practical guide for health professionals / Jonathan C. Smith.
        p.   cm.
    Includes bibliographical references.
    ISBN 0-8261-1282-X (hardcover)
    1. Relaxation.   I. Title.
    BF637.R45S55   1999
    613.7'9—dc21   99-21027
                                                                           CIP

Printed in the United States of America

Larry McKeon
Friend, Colleague, Pioneer

Contents

List of Tables

1

ABC Relaxation Theory in a Nutshell

This is a book about relaxation. But let me begin by sharing a story that at first glance might seem out of place. It is a remarkable image from modern astronomy, one I use as an introduction in most of my relaxation seminars. I believe it captures the essence of what relaxation is all about.

One of the most important events in space science has been the launching of the Hubble telescope. Ten times more powerful than any telescope on earth, the orbiting Hubble can see where no one has seen before. Two things make the Hubble an especially powerful tool. First, it can examine the heavens in the utter silence of space, undistracted by the city lights, haze, and noise of earth. Second, the Hubble can sustain its focus, unmoved, for hours, days, and even weeks. No earth telescope can do this—shifting continents, passing traffic, changes in the atmosphere, and the rotation of the planet itself mean that the gaze of any land-based telescope is never perfectly steady.

For 10 days in late 1995, astronomers conducted an experiment that changed our vision of the universe. It was a study that had never and indeed could never have been conducted before. In the "deep field experiment," astronomers aimed the Hubble toward a patch of space that has always appeared completely empty, a small dark spot of sky where earth telescopes indicated that nothing existed. (For stargazers, this empty area is close to the handle of the "Big Dipper" and is about one-hundredth the size of the moon.) What really exists in this empty space? After a full 2 weeks of sustained, unmoving focus, the Hubble had a surprising answer: 1 trillion stars, extending to the very edge of the universe—thousands of galaxies, each containing billions of stars. Astronomers have concluded that this discovery transforms our vision of the universe. It is far richer than anyone ever imagined. The deep field experiment shows that what we thought was empty space is filled with an unimaginable richness of stars. And the key to this discovery was sustained, passive, simple focus. This, as we shall see, is also the key to relaxation.

DOWN TO EARTH: ABC RELAXATION TRAINING

Relaxation is often taught as a mechanical health chore, something done at the clinic (yoga center, gym, health class) and left behind. In this book I suggest that relaxation can be much more, a journey into inner space with potential for adventure and discovery. This is true not only for approaches such as meditation, imagery, and yoga, which are deeply embedded in religion and philosophy, but also such ordinary tools of our trade as progressive muscle relaxation (PMR) and autogenic training (AT).

I call my approach attentional behavioral cognitive (or ABC) relaxation training. We begin with a simple idea. The key to relaxation is sustaining *a*ttention while diminishing overt *b*ehavior and covert or *c*ognitive activity. To elaborate, all forms of relaxation, both secular and spiritual, involve the basic attentional act of *sustaining passive simple focusing*. To understand, we need to consider a few down-to-earth facts of life.

Life is effortful. We strive to achieve our daily goals, anticipate our future, and reflect on our past. Life is discursive, or moving and changing (from the Latin for "moving to and fro"). We plan schedules, vacations, and shopping lists. And when the discursive efforts of life take their toll—wear and tear on body, mind, and soul—we relax. We let go and cease active, goal-directed planning, effort, and appraisal. We focus on just one simple thing. Relaxation is sustained passive simple focus.

Everyone has experienced special moments of passive simple focus. One might gaze at a sunset and for an instant feel a sense of peace and beauty as golden rays burst through violet clouds. Or after reading a moving story, one might close one's eyes and savor the moment, feeling distant and far away from the cares of the world. Throughout life, all of us spontaneously encounter a rich variety of instances of passive simple focus through music, poetry, art, prayer, and so on. Such moments are part of life's treasures; but such moments come and go quickly. The sun sets. The music ends. The poem is finished. We go on with our day's work. The secret of relaxation training is to sustain the moment. This is a very difficult thing to do, like balancing a basketball on a calm and steady fingertip. *Sustaining*, uninterrupted, the state of passive simple focus is made easier by practicing a formal relaxation technique. And our research has discovered that, like the Hubble telescope, such sustained focus can have its rewards and surprises.

The Cycle of Renewal

All approaches to relaxation evoke a fundamental process of healing and growth in which one withdraws from the efforts of the day, recovers, and opens up to the world. I call this the Cycle of Renewal. The idea of a cyclical renewal process has been around for several millennia and can be manifest at many levels. World religions speak of global cycles of death and rebirth, repentance and forgiveness, as well as acceptance and enlightenment. Professional approaches to relaxation involve mastering the discipline of withdrawing from everyday stress for healing and recovery, and returning to the world refreshed and restored. And each time we pause and sigh we display a moment of relaxation and renewal.

ABC Relaxation Theory presents a universal, evidence-based lexicon of relaxation and renewal and proposes how the cycle of renewal works. Our lexicon consists of three basic constructs: relaxation states (R-States), relaxation beliefs (R-Beliefs), and relaxation attitudes (R-Attitudes). R-States, R-Beliefs, and R-Attitudes determine the effectiveness of all of relaxation.

R-States

A decade of research (Smith, 1999), involving several thousand participants, has revealed that relaxation evokes at least nine special states of mind, which I term *R-*(Relaxation) *States:*

- Sleepiness (feeling "drowsy, napping").
- Disengagement (feeling "distant, far away, indifferent").
- Physical Relaxation (feeling "physically limp, warm, and heavy").
- Mental Quiet ("Mind is silent, quiet, free of thought").
- Mental Relaxation (feeling "at ease, peaceful").
- Strength and Awareness (feeling "energized, confident, focused, clear, aware").
- Joy (feeling "happy, joyful; having fun").
- Love and Thankfulness (feeling "love for others, generally thankful").
- Prayerfulness (feeling "spiritual, reverent, prayerful").

R-States are more than the rewards of relaxation; they are what make relaxation work. If an exercise does not evoke an appropriate set of R-States, it will have little effect.

An Illustration of R-States and Relaxation

We can better understand the role of R-States in relaxation if we take a close look at a (hypothetical) relaxation case study, that of someone who experienced a simple and familiar relaxation activity—a vacation.

> *Joan is an accountant. She works long and hard and lives under high levels of chronic stress—client deadlines, complex reports, budgets, phone calls, and so on. Joan decides to take a week off and take a bike ride to a nearby mountain retreat. The night before, she retires to bed and experiences the first R-State,* Sleepiness. *The next day, she packs her gear, gets on her bike, and begins her journey on a nearby path in the park. After about half an hour, Joan reaches a wooded retreat. She looks back and sees her hometown in the distance. She sighs, very glad that her home and hectic work are beginning to feel like faraway memories. She experiences the R-State* Disengagement. *After a day of riding, Joan reaches a camping spot. She puts her bike away and sits on a soft patch of grass. She stretches, lies down, and closes her eyes. Her mind is still, without thought. She experiences* Mental Quiet. *Her body feels wonderfully relaxed, "loose and limp." She has a nice sensation of "sinking" in the soft grass. Joan feels* Physical Relaxation. *After about 15 minutes, Joan begins to notice how calm and peaceful her mind feels. She is now truly at ease, safe from the world of conflict and confrontation. This is* Mental Relaxation. *Free from her conflicts at work and home, Joan opens her eyes, notices how refreshed and renewed she feels. She is focused and clear. This is* Strength and Awareness.*
>
> *The pressures of the day a distant memory, her body relaxed, and mind calm and clear, Joan can begin to see clearly the sky above and the trees around. She is struck with their beauty and wonder. She feels a sense of deep harmony with the world. She feels* Joy. *Joan savors the beauty of the moment, feeling the R-State* Love and Thankfulness. *She is grateful that she has had the opportunity to experience this special moment and wishes her friends were there to share it with her. In time, evening approaches. The air grows quiet. Joan gazes at the sky above and sees the emergence with the first evening star in the vast heavens. And for an instant, Joan is struck with a sense of awe and wonder of the deep world around. Joan experiences a moment of* Prayerfulness.

Joan experienced all of our nine R-States. Many clients do not. Each R-State is quite possibly powerful in and of itself. It is important to keep in mind that what enabled Joan to experience this remarkable universe of relaxation was the attentional act of *sustaining passive simple focus*—the same thing that enabled the Hubble telescope to see the edge of the universe. Many hikers never experience Disengagement, Mental Relaxation, or Joy. Joan did because she became *passive for a sustained period of time* and let go of all unnecessary deliberate, planful effort. She chose not to spend her time effortfully planning budgets, schedules, and accounts. And she chose not to turn her ride into a race against time or a competitive challenge (perhaps to discover as many wild birds as possible, cover as much ground as possible, or meet some precise itinerary). Joan simply let go and enjoyed the hike. In addition, Joan's *focus was simple*—just riding a bike, appreciating a wooded park, enjoying a campsite, feeling the soft grass, and gazing into the night sky.

R-States are what make all of relaxation work. Different approaches to relaxation may evoke different R-States. And different R-States may be best for different clinical goals. Preliminary research (Smith, Amutio, Anderson, & Aria, 1996; Smith, 1999) suggests that the tense–let go cycles of PMR seem to be conducive to Disengagement (feeling "distant, far away, indifferent") and Physical Relaxation. In contrast, hatha yoga stretches seem to evoke feelings of Strength and Awareness. Imagery tends to cultivate feelings of Joy. However, this is indeed a new world of relaxation, one with little research (see Smith, 1999). Rather than look for strict formulas, this book suggests a more cautious approach: determine which R-States are desired by a client and, through trial and error, which combinations of techniques seem to be most effective for evoking these R-States. For example, a highly anxious client might want to learn to Disengage from anxiety-arousing negative thinking and may discover that meditation and breathing work best at evoking Disengagement. A depressed client may want a technique that fosters feelings of Strength and Awareness as well as Mental Relaxation. She may discover that a combination of PMR and imagery works best. See various approaches in Table 1.1 at end of chapter.

R-Beliefs

Our thoughts and opinions about relaxation can have a profound impact on the course of relaxation training. ABC Relaxation Theory identifies two groups of relaxation cognitions: Relaxation attitudes (R-Attitudes) are negative thoughts that contribute to avoiding relaxation or prematurely abandoning a relaxation program ("Relaxation is laziness," "relaxation is hypnosis"). Relaxation beliefs (R-Beliefs) are somewhat philosophical perspectives conducive to deeper and more generalized relaxation. Currently research identifies 8 R-Beliefs:

- Optimism ("View the world with optimism.")
- Acceptance ("Accept things that cannot be changed.")
- Honesty ("Be honest with yourself and others.")
- Taking It Easy ("Know when to let go and take it easy.")
- Love ("Relate to others with love and compassion.")
- Inner Wisdom ("Trust the healing wisdom of the body.")
- God ("Trust God's love and guidance.")
- Deeper Perspective ("Put your concerns in deeper perspective.")

ABC Relaxation Training does not stop with the instruction of techniques. The second major task is addressing a client's attitudes and beliefs through cognitive restructuring, a central feature of cognitive-behavior therapy. In ABC Relaxation Training, the goal of cognitive restructuring is to identify and reduce irrational and maladaptive attitudes that may inhibit relaxation and foster the development of rational and adaptive beliefs conducive to the practice of relaxation and the generalization of R-States to life at large.

In summary, the overall goal of ABC Relaxation Training can be put in terms of a simple formula. Traditional relaxation is often presented in stimulus-response (S-R) terms, in which the stimulus of a relaxation technique produces the response of various relaxation benefits:

RELAXATION TECHNIQUE

↓

RELAXATION BENEFITS

In ABC Relaxation Training, technique practice evokes the Cycle of Renewal, which in turn mediates desired relaxation outcomes. Specifically, R-States, R-Beliefs, and R-Attitudes interact and contribute to improvements in health, performance, and well-being associated with relaxation.

RELAXATION TECHNIQUE

↕

R-BELIEFS/ATTITUDES ↔ R-STATES

↕

RELAXATION BENEFITS

TRAINING FORMATS

For nearly 20 years I have taught relaxation to several thousand individuals, and my students have taught many more. Originally, I would present a menu of at least five approaches (Smith, 1987), expecting clients to select a single, favored technique. My bias had been that people would gravitate toward a single approach, PMR, yoga, breathing, imagery, or meditation. Instead, my clients have taught me an important lesson. Over 95% prefer a combination from at least five different approaches. Almost all clients prefer highly individualized relaxation training, one that expresses not only their interests, but their deepest beliefs. In this way, teaching relaxation most resembles the highly fluid and individualized goals of psychotherapy and counseling, especially *multimodal behavior therapy* (Lazarus, 1976, 1997). ABC Relaxation Training attempts to meet this ideal by presenting exercises in three steps:

1. *Preliminary training.* Begin by teaching a client not one but five or six approaches to relaxation (PMR, AT, breathing exercises, yoga stretching, imagery, and meditation). Make sure to teach "purified" versions of each approach so that clients can identify the unique relaxation effects of each.
2. *Exercise selection.* With the client, select which specific exercises seem to work best.
3. *Program development.* Fashion exercises, words suggestive of desired relaxation states (R-States), and affirmations of relaxation-supportive beliefs (R-Beliefs) into a personal practice program that has both clinical and aesthetic integrity.

In the following chapters I present the procedural specifics of my approach. The reader will quickly discover that my approach is fully compatible with what he or she may already practice. Indeed, this book works fine for practitioners who, for whatever reason, have chosen to specialize in one technique, whether PMR, self-hypnosis, prayer, or yoga.

ABC Relaxation Training suggests four individualized training formats, which can be deployed separately or together: the Grand Tours of relaxation (chapter 2), specific technique instruction for six major professional approaches to relaxation (chapter 3), scripting (chapter 4), and brief relaxation training (chapter 5).

The Grand Tours of Relaxation

Prospective clients and practitioners are often misinformed about the nature of relaxation. Common misconceptions include the view that relaxation is nothing more than a relaxation response and that casual everyday activities are the same as professional relaxation. One of the first steps in ABC Relaxation Training is to provide an orientation as to the nature of the program. Proper preparation orients the client as to the nature of relaxation training, enhances realistic expectations and motivation, reviews possible goals and problems, and assesses relaxation skill deficiencies and possible technique selection. When presented alone, preparation activities can effectively educate potential clients as to the nature and potential of relaxation.

The Grand Tours of Relaxation introduce ABC Relaxation Theory and the six major approaches to professional relaxation training. The Grand Tour lecture focuses on basic concepts. The Grand Tour workshop demonstrates four groups of exercises: (1) PMR and AT (which tend to foster the R-States Sleep, Disengagement, and Physical Relaxation); (2) yoga stretching and breathing (for Strength and Awareness as well as Mental Relaxation; (3) imagery (Joy); and (4) meditation (Mental Quiet and Prayerfulness). Clients discuss and select which exercises work best. The overall objective is to enable participants to discover that different relaxation techniques evoke different R-States and work for different people.

Specific Technique Instruction

This book presents fairly traditional instructions to six major approaches to professional relaxation. However, ABC Relaxation Training deviates from tradition in two important ways. At no point do we claim that a technique is the only, most effective, or best approach. If a technique does not work, our tendency is not to stick with it and introduce modifications; instead, the trainer tries other approaches until the client finds what works. In addition, we attempt to teach relatively "pure" versions of techniques (for PMR, "tensing and letting go" are not mixed with stretching, breathing, or imagery) so that clients can discover the unique R-States associated with each technique.

Relaxation Scripting

Relaxation scripting involves taking preferred client exercises and exercise elements and crafting a relaxation script or tape tailored to client needs. Hundreds of relaxation tapes are available through bookstores and health clubs. However, each suffers from a serious problem. Lack of individualization risks exposing clients to exercises that are not suited for them and indeed may pose problems. In contrast, relaxation scripting is highly individualized. After several weeks of training in at least five approaches, the client and trainer select desired exercises and exercise components and identify a preferred order of presentation. Next, client and trainer add a variety of deepening enhancements, including words and phrases suggesting various R-States and R-Beliefs. The product is a relaxation tape that is something of a work of art, specifically designed for the client.

Brief Relaxation Training

Brief relaxation training (BRT) is an accelerated approach to ABC Relaxation Training in which a trainer demonstrates the major approaches to relaxation and crafts a client relaxation sequence in a single 60-minute session. Presenting BRT requires considerable skill. The trainer must first demonstrate a variety of sample exercises and continuously monitor client preferences through nonverbal cues. Using such cues, one continuously modifies instruction, adding and deleting exercises and navigating through those that appear to work best. At the end of the session, the trainer has identified a desired sequence of exercises and exercise enhancements for the client and is ready to record an individualized relaxation tape.

TABLE 1.1 Comparison of Examples from Six Major Approaches to Relaxation

Approach	Simple Focal Stimulus	Passivity	How Sustained
Progressive muscle relaxation	Sensations of muscle tension and release of tension	Deliberately letting go of tension after tensing up	A series of tense–let go exercises is presented, moving throughout the entire body; the instructor maintains instructional talk or "patter"
Autogenic training	Physically relaxing phrases such as "Hands and arms are warm and heavy"	Any effort to deliberately conjure up feelings of warmth and heaviness should be avoided; one repeats phrases with "utter indifference."	Client repeats phrases over and over, like an endless echo.
Breathing exercises	The flow of breath with every inhalation and exhalation	Breathing without force or effort	Practicing a sequence of several breathing exercises
Yoga stretching	Sensations from joints, ligaments, and muscles as they are stretched and unstretched	One must not "force" a stretch but do it gently and gracefully.	One does a sequence of stretches.
Imagery	A pleasing, relaxing image, involving all the senses (e.g., a vacation spot)	One is the passive observer and does not actively and deliberately "direct" the image, like a movie director.	The complex evolution of the image sustains attention.
Meditation	One attends to an utterly simple stimulus, like a mantra or candle flame.	Any thought or effort other than the simple sustaining of attention is to be avoided.	Difficult to sustain attention

2

Preparing for Relaxation: The Grand Tours and Assessment

The first step in teaching relaxation is to prepare the client. This involves two steps: (1) presenting introductory orientation information and (2) assessing client needs, desires, and special problems. Such preparation helps the client and trainer articulate appropriate relaxation goals, select exercises, and most important, establish proper expectations. Clients, as well as more than a few health professionals, often approach training with misconceptions. Some may accept the relaxation response perspective that all approaches have the same effect. Others, encouraged by overstated media presentations of miracle cures, may expect immediate dramatic results. And many may expect little, believing that relaxation is little more than taking a nap. Preparation can do much to foster realistic perceptions about the promise and limitations of relaxation.

ORIENTING THE CLIENT

The Grand Tour of Relaxation is perhaps one of the most useful innovations of this book. Two versions introduce and demonstrate the key concepts of ABC Relaxation Theory and ABC Relaxation Training, one a didactic lecture, the other an experiential workshop with practical exercises.

The Grand Tour Lecture

The Grand Tour lecture is a 90-minute talk on ABC relaxation theory and training. The lecture begins with a review of traditional views of relaxation. The key idea is that relaxation innovations have typically been presented "top down," from a religious figure, a guru, a physician, or a psychologist. In contrast, ABC Relaxation Theory is based on scientific evidence coming from the "ground up," reflecting the "wisdom of a thousand voices." The basic hypotheses of ABC Relaxation Theory are then presented: (1) different approaches to relaxation have different effects and work for different people, and (2) all relaxation techniques work by evoking specific R-States, supported through R-Beliefs. The lecture concludes with a discussion of R-States participants have experienced in a recent relaxation activity. Precise verbatim script instructions are presented in Table 2.1 at the end of this chapter.

The Grand Tour Workshop

The Grand Tour workshop is a 90-minute experiential seminar that presents samples from each of the six major approaches to relaxation. Clients explore what I have found to be highly accessible and interesting representative exercises from progressive muscle relaxation (PMR), autogenic "warmth/heaviness" exercises, active yoga stretching, passive breathing exercises, imagery, and meditation. In addition, the Grand Tour introduces R-States as well as the multidimensional nature of relaxation effects.

The Grand Tour workshop can be presented individually or to groups. First, the trainer introduces ABC Relaxation Theory with the notion of R-States. He or she presents instructions for all techniques. After each set of exercises, clients are asked to report their R-States through a nonintrusive signal system ("Raise your right index finger if you experience this R-State"). When all exercises are presented, the trainer discusses client reactions. Useful probe questions include the following:

> "Which exercises did you like, and dislike? Why?"
> "Did you notice any differences among exercises? What were they?"
> "Which R-States did you experience?"
> "What might be some of the specific effects of specific exercises?"
> "What might be some of the uses of different R-States?"

It is important to tailor the grand tour to the client or client group. I suggest tour modifications for five populations: (1) achievement-oriented clients potentially hostile to relaxation training, (2) clients considering relaxation for health maintenance or to facilitate recovery, (3) substance abuse clients, (4) clients interested in spiritually oriented meditation, and

(5) clients interested in relaxation as an approach for enhancing prayer or worship in their practice of religion. Precise verbatim script instructions are presented in Table 2.2 at the end of this chapter.

THE FORMAL ASSESSMENT OF RELAXATION

It is not enough to present a relaxation exercise and assume a client is relaxed. Often exercises do not work or need adjusting. Formal assessment tools facilitate the process of determining the effectiveness of relaxation training. Assessment options include biofeedback equipment (not considered in this volume), behavioral observation, verbal report, and psychological assessment.

Behavioral Assessment

Behavioral observation is the least intrusive way to measure relaxation. (For an excellent review of behavioral assessment of relaxation, see Poppen, 1998). It is valuable for assessing overall level of physiological arousal and perhaps less useful for measuring R-States, R-Beliefs, or R-Attitudes. The Behavioral Signs of Relaxation Rating Scale focuses on three types of readily observable behavior indicative of relaxation: breathing, posture, and movement (Table 2.3 at end of chapter).

Breathing

A variety of breathing behaviors can indicate deepened relaxation. Most generally, breathing that is rapid and jerky (with gasping or holding breath) and involves movement of the chest suggests arousal. When breathing becomes slower and more even, with greater use of the diaphragm (indicated by a slowly rising and falling stomach), one can infer deepened relaxation.

Posture

It is fairly easy to observe a client's posture during relaxation, and it is useful to differentiate postures associated with tension as opposed to Disengagement and Physical Relaxation. These R-States may be reflected by such postures as slightly sloped shoulders, slightly tilted head, and a general openness of jaws, palms, fingers, knees, and feet. Jaws may be slightly parted; palms open; fingers curled, not straight or clenched, and knees and feet pointing apart. In exercises emphasizing opening up (yoga, breathing, and some meditation), neck and back are more likely to be calmly, not rigidly, erect. It is as if each vertebra were precisely stacked so that no effort is needed to keep the back and neck erect. Also, a yoga practitioner should execute and maintain a stretch or posture slowly and smoothly without jerks or effort.

Movement

Skeletal muscle activity is a sign of muscle tension. Movement can be voluntary (blinking, open eyes, looking around, chewing, biting lips, swallowing, clenching, bracing) or involuntary (twitching, tics). Often, skin smoothness can indicate level of muscle tension (furrowed brow, bulging muscles).

A variety of subtle nonverbal cues may suggest various R-States. Some are relatively direct. Most people can recognize the behavioral signs of Sleepiness (nodding, deep breathing, etc.). Physical Relaxation may be reflected by the behavioral signs just outlined. Obviously, a smile suggests Joy. Considerable empathic skill may be required to detect Disengagement, Mental Quiet, Mental Relaxation, Strength and Awareness, Love and Thankfulness, and Prayerfulness. For these, a trainer may have to resort to verbal communication.

Psychological Assessment

Symptom and Arousal Reduction

Traditionally relaxation assessment is limited to identification of high specific and localized target symptoms, for example:

Breathing difficulties

Foot pain

Lower back pain

Neck tension

Shoulder tension

Stomach distress

Wrist and elbow pain (from typing, writing, etc.)

Several hundred assessment tools are available for measuring stress arousal and arousal-related symptoms (Derogatis & Coons, 1993); it is beyond the scope of this book to note them all. I have found two multidimensional inventories to be particularly useful: the Derogatis Stress Profile (DSP) and the SCL-90-R (Derogatis & Coons, 1993). The DSP taps three external stimulus dimensions of stress (job, home, health); five personal attributes and coping measures (time pressure; driven behavior, or the compulsive need to be constantly involved in constructive behavior; attitude posture, or an aspect of the achievement ethic; relaxation potential, or the potential for healthy diversion; and role definition, or the expectation that one bears sole responsibility for dealing with the demands of life); and three symptom measures (aggression-hostility, tension-anxiety, and depression).

The SCL-90-R and its brief cousin, the Brief Symptom Inventory, tap nine primary symptom dimensions: somatization, obsessive-compulsive symptoms, interpersonal sensitivity, depression, anxiety, hostility, phobic anxiety, paranoid ideation, and psychoticism.

Several unidimensional arousal and symptom scales have particular relevance for relaxation training and may provide a more sensitive assessment than multidimensional inventories: the Beck Depression Inventory (Beck, Ward, Mendelson, Mock, & Erbaugh, 1961), the State-Trait Anxiety Inventory (Spielberger, Gorsuch, & Lushene, 1970), the Center for Epidemiologic Studies Depression Scales (Radloff, 1977), and the Profile of Mood States (McNair, Lorr, & Dropplemann, 1971). (*See* Table 2.4 at end of chapter.)

Smith Relaxation Inventories

ABC Relaxation Theory suggests that the assessment of relaxation go beyond measurement of arousal during the training session, or symptom reduction when the session is over. Relaxation is a rich and complex task; we serve our clients best when we attempt to understand all facets of their journeys.

A client brings to a relaxation session a history of beliefs and experiences. Some R-Beliefs may facilitate the mastery of relaxation, while others may interfere. For ABC relaxation, part of the task of training involves cognitive restructuring, that is, identifying, reinforcing, and modifying beliefs and attitudes when appropriate. To this end, I have developed two inventories, modestly named the Smith Relaxation Beliefs Inventory (SRBI), which taps beliefs supportive of relaxation, and the Smith Relaxation Attitudes Inventory (SRAI), which taps attitudes that interfere with relaxation.

Furthermore, most clients already know something about relaxation and have discovered R-States and casual activities they prefer. A skilled relaxation trainer can capitalize on this history by introducing formal techniques tailored to a preferred family of relaxation activity; ability to sustain passive, simple focus; and capacity to experience specific R-States. For example, a client may prefer the causal activities of dance and walking (movement/posture family activities), have little capacity to sustain passive simple focus, and report feelings of Strength and Awareness when relaxing. Using behavioral shaping (beginning with easy, familiar versions of techniques), a trainer might begin with simple yoga stretching, an approach from the movement/posture family that appears to foster Strength and Awareness and (at simple levels) calls for little sustained passive simple focusing.

Similarly, once a formal relaxation strategy has been selected, trainer and client can select casual relaxation activities that reinforce targeted states. For example, if training focuses on progressive muscle relaxation and autogenic training as means to evoke Physical Relaxation and Disengagement, one might suggest additional activities from the somatic/emotional family that may have the same effect, perhaps massage, steam baths, and sunbathing when appropriate. Assessment of relaxation history can be assisted through my Smith Recalled Relaxation Activities Inventory (SRRAI), a test that asks clients to describe how they already relax, and what R-States they already experience.

It is also useful to know what R-States a client generally experiences and what he or she desires from relaxation. The Smith Relaxation Dispositions/ Motivations Inventory (SRDMI) taps R-States at a dispositional (or "trait") level, in other words, how generally relaxed (for each R-State) a client is throughout the course of a two-week period. The same inventory measures a client's R-Motivations, or desire to experience more of any particular R-State. Finally the Smith Relaxation Concerns Inventory (SRCI) taps those problems and goals clients claim most readily respond to relaxation (managing pain, improving performance, etc.). As such, the SRCI can be used as a clinical screening and outcome measure.

Relaxation training has immediate and delayed reinforcements, short-term, intermediate, and long-term outcomes. A client may during a session experience rewarding reductions in stress and increments in specific R-States. These reinforcements can be assessed through the Smith Relaxation States Inventory (SRSI). In time, he or she may experience intermediate and long-term changes in all aspects of relaxation, including desired R-States (SRDMI), R-State dispositions (SRDMI), targeted problem concerns and goals (SRCI), attitudes resistant to relaxation (SRAI), beliefs supportive of relaxation (SRBI), and casual everyday activities that reinforce relaxation outside the practice session (SRRAI).

In sum, a comprehensive understanding of relaxation must examine a variety of dimensions. As we shall see, relaxation research is beginning to provide insights as to how these variables are interrelated. The Smith Relaxation Inventory Series is available through Springer Publishing Company. Recent versions of actual inventories are in the Appendix.

Verbal Report

Another relatively simple approach to relaxation assessment is to listen to spontaneous client reports. In addition to providing overall appraisals of their techniques ("This technique worked very well," "The second technique did not work"), client choice of words can reveal underlying relaxation processes. For example, clients who report feeling "limp" or "loose" are obviously describing Physical Relaxation. Those who feel "indifferent" or "forgetting" are describing Disengagement. If a client uses words that do not appear on our word lists, one can look for similarities. For example, feeling "limber" most resembles words listed for physical relaxation; "in my own space" resembles Disengagement, "unburdened" resembles Mental Relaxation, and so on. See Table 2.5 at end of chapter for an extended listing of words associated with various R-States.

Finger Signal System

I have found it useful to assess R-States through a signal system. In the simple version, a trainer slowly and briefly describes each R-State and asks clients to raise the right finger whenever they hear an R-State they experience. In a more complete version, a client is given something of a "4-point finger/hand Likert scale." A client raises the right index finger to indicate that he or she is experiencing "a little" of the described R-State. Both left and right fingers indicate one is "moderately" experiencing an R-State. Raising the right hand indicates that one is experiencing an R-State "very much." Raising nothing indicates that an R-State is not experienced. *See* Table 2.6 at end of chapter.

ASSESSMENT TOPICS

Armed with biofeedback, behavioral, and psychological assessment tools, the relaxation trainer is ready to acquire a complete and full understanding of the client's relaxation needs and assets. A variety of topics should be considered.

Assessment of Possible Problems

On rare occasions relaxation exercises can have unwanted physical effects. Although relaxation is comfortable and safe for most people, some physical exercises present a level of risk perhaps comparable to that of a mild exercise program, such as walking for 20 minutes or climbing four flights of stairs. Most important, clients should stop practicing and consult a physician if they experience any of the following possible cardiac symptoms:

Pain or tightness in the chest
Irregular heartbeat
Extreme shortness of breath
Feeling light-headed, nauseous, or dizzy (these can also be associated with breathing exercises)

Clients under treatment for any medical condition should inform their physicians of the nature of the relaxation exercises they plan to practice. Precautions for specific techniques are listed in a later chapter. A trainer can present this list to clients or their physicians.

Relaxation training can alter the required dosage levels for prescription medication, particularly for patients undergoing treatment for hypertension, diabetes, depression, anxiety, and any disorder influenced by changes in general metabolic rate. Although the potential for risk has not been consistently demonstrated, the state of relaxation itself is frequently associated with changes in general metabolic rate. As a result, need for medication may decrease (and in a few paradoxical cases temporarily increase).

If clients report any physical symptom associated with a specific organ, joint, or muscle group, exercises targeted to this group should generally be avoided (unless part of a supervised rehabilitation program). Caution should be taken for clients displaying or reporting injury or recent surgery, pregnancy, weakness, or illness.

Relaxation Treatment Goals

Occasionally, clients desire relaxation to treat highly specific and localized target symptoms, for example, earlier we have noted:

Breathing difficulties

Foot pain

Lower back pain

Neck tension

Shoulder tension

Stomach distress

Wrist and elbow pain

Clients often can identify such difficulties with little assistance. Here, treatment might include specific exercises from PMR, AT, yoga stretching, or breathing matched to the symptom (e.g., shoulder tension–shoulder PMR tense/release cycle) and, time and resources permitting, supplemented by the multi-technique approach of this book.

Our research (Smith, in press) has determined that most clients (nearly 75%) relax to manage stress, particularly frustration, worry, anxiety, and depression. Nearly half relax to enhance sleep and health. Spiritual and psychological growth are the third most popular objectives, claimed by over a third. More specifically, factor analysis reveals nine claimed relaxation benefits: Medical Benefits (preparing and recovering from surgery and dental procedures; coping with medications); Substance Abuse, Psychological Distress, Sleep and Pain, Interpersonal Stress, General health, Creativity, Spirituality, and Athletics. These are assessed in Smith Relaxation Concerns Inventory (Appendix).

Once clients are introduced to the notion of R-States, R-Beliefs, and R-Attitudes, they may express treatment goals in terms of these dimensions (e.g., "I want to feel more Strengthened and Aware, be more Optimistic, or have a more open attitude about the possibilities of relaxation"). For a script for assessing relaxation goals, see Table 2.7 (end of chapter).

WHEN TO ASSESS RELAXATION

Trainers and researchers who wish to assess relaxation have several options as to when to test.

Within-Session Effects

Most relaxation researchers recognize the importance of evaluating level of relaxation within a session. Somatic relaxation is relatively easy to assess with biofeedback equipment. However, how does one assess R-States before a session is over? There are two options. First, interrupt a session and ask for an immediate assessment of how one felt at the moment of interruption. Or one might use the recalled session approach.

Immediately Recalled Session Effects

At the end of a session, one asks clients to *recall* how they felt during the session. Researchers often make the mistake of assuming that immediate postsession assessment automatically measures what transpired during a session. Unless subjects are asked to recall how they felt, postsession assessment often measures aftereffects.

Immediate Aftereffects

When considering the impact of a relaxation session, it is important to assess both within-session effects and effects immediate after session termination. Often they might be quite different. A client might find 30 minutes of imagery or meditation not particularly rewarding and yet feel deeply refreshed and invigorated immediately after. Noting such aftereffects can help reinforce practice by reassuring a client that a technique is working.

Recalled Typical Recent Session Effect

A useful way of assessing a client's potential for R-States is to ask him or her to recall a typical relaxation activity completed in the past week or two and describe the effects of this activity. Much of the early research on ABC Theory has used this approach.

Day Effects

Clients often recognize the impact of a day's relaxation session when the day is over. For example, a morning practice session may in itself be relatively uneventful. A client might report that the usually hectic commute home from work didn't seem so bad. Day's end can be an ideal time to reflect on the day's events and identify unexpected relaxation effects.

Situational Effects

Often clients learn to relax in order to master a specific problem, for example, public speaking anxiety, distress related to medical procedures, and so on. By identifying a target problem situation ahead of time, a client can determine the impact of relaxation on this situation.

Long-term Dispositional Effects

Relaxation can have a long-term effect on an enduring psychological predisposition or trait—for example, anxiety or depression. A popular format for trait questionnaires is to preface items with the instruction "Please rate how you generally or typically feel." It is my suspicion that when applied to R-States, respondents in fact are rating how they felt for the past week or two.

Care must be taken in assessing the subjective effects of relaxation. Just what is it one wants to measure? The immediate effects or the aftereffects of a specific session? How relaxed one generally is? Or one's capacity for evoking a relaxation effect? Different questions can yield quite different answers with different implications. For example, a client may experience Disengagement at different times, including during a session, immediately after a session, all the time, prior to a stressful encounter, or "on demand," whenever desired. The capacity to Disengage during select relaxation sessions may well be healthy; however, chronic Disengagement could well reflect depersonalization disorder.

RELAXATION DIARIES AND RECORD SHEETS

A comprehensive assessment of relaxation might include a week of daily record taking, in which a client indicates what R-States and stress symptoms were encountered throughout the day, their antecedent stimuli, and reinforcing consequences. Such assessment can enable a relaxation trainer to determine which R-States a client already has some skill at evoking. Generally, when teaching relaxation, it is desirable to make the task of mastering a new technique as easy as possible. If a client already knows how to Disengage and experience some Physical Relaxation, I recommend starting with techniques that tend to evoke these same R-States (PMR and AT). Daily records and diaries also can determine if certain R-States emerge at certain times of day, perhaps reflecting a circadian rhythm.

Training could be fashioned after patterns that have been determined. For example, if a client wishes to master yogaform stretching and breathing exercises in order to evoke the R-States Strength and Awareness and Mental Relaxation, and he or she is most likely to experience these states early in the morning, then early morning would be the appropriate time to learn stretching and breathing. Once mastered, relaxation techniques can be used in more challenging circumstances, say prior to a stressful encounter. Unfortunately, diaries and records, no matter how desirable in principle, are usually not feasible in an age of time-limited care.

SELECTING A TIME AND PLACE TO PRACTICE

One of the most difficult tasks of relaxation training is to teach a client to practice regularly. Our research clearly shows that daily practice is perhaps the most important predictor of success at relaxation, even more important than level of pathology, anxiety, or number of years one has practiced a technique. I suggest using behavioral shaping to foster regularity of practice (Smith, 1986). The most important step is selecting a practice time and place.

1. Brainstorm possible practice times and places. Relaxation settings should be relatively quiet, comfortable, and convenient.
2. Select a preferred time and place each day. Clients may have to vary practice times and places in order to maintain a practice schedule.
3. Try to identify potential unforseen problems with selected practice times and places. Play "devil's advocate" and try to figure out how the tentatively selected schedule will fail.
4. Modify time and place to accommodate problems.
5. Assign the client to try out the tentative schedule using a pleasant, passive relaxing activity, rather than a professional technique. That is, for the first week, a client may spend a half hour before bedtime reading pleasant nonfiction. It is important that the "time off activity" be something the client already finds pleasant and rewarding. The purpose of this step is to reinforce the habit of taking time aside for relaxation. Once this habit is established, relaxation training can begin.

ASSESSMENT AND THE EIGHT
MAJOR QUESTIONS: SUMMARY

Before teaching relaxation to a client, a trainer should have answers to the following preliminary questions:

1. **Goals.** *Why does my client want to learn relaxation? What R-States and R-Beliefs does he/she desire? What specific goals does he/she have?*
2. **Relaxation and other treatment/training objectives.** *How can I integrate relaxation into whatever other treatment my client is receiving (psychotherapy, counseling, medical treatment, rehabilitation, exercise programs, religious ceremony and prayer, creative performance, and sports)? Some treatment interventions (such as classical desensitization, stress inoculation training, and anger management) have clearly specified how and when relaxation should be introduced. Unfortunately, for other treatment and training programs, the trainer must rely on his or her professional judgement. Hopefully the ideas of this book will provide some clues.*
3. **Casual relaxation (and possible technique preferences).** *What casual relaxation activities does my client already engage in? Are these similar to any formal relaxation technique, both in terms of relaxation family and R-State evoked? Can these be woven into a relaxation program?*
4. **R-Dispositions.** *What R-Dispositions does my client generally report? What techniques may facilitate these dispositions? Is it desirable to teach techniques that augment dispositions already present, or dispositions that go beyond what the client already experiences?*
5. **R-Attitudes.** *What attitudes does my client have that may interfere with relaxation? How might I as a trainer address these negative attitudes? Are there any specific techniques my client clearly does not want?*
6. **R-Beliefs.** *What beliefs does my client have that may enhance or deepen relaxation? Are there any techniques these beliefs may facilitate?*
7. **Problems.** *Does my client have any specific medical problems that may interfere with relaxation training? If so, what exercises should be avoided or presented with caution?*
8. **Logistics.** *Can my client develop a realistic relaxation practice schedule? Has he/she successfully completed a week of "taking time aside" for relaxation.*

Once training begins, a trainer should continuously consider the following process questions.

1. **Goals.** *To what extent is my client reporting improvement on selected relaxation objectives?*
2. **Integrating relaxation with other treatments and training programs.** *If my client is currently in some other treatment or training program, how can I integrate current program processes and objectives?*

3. **Casual relaxation.** *What casual relaxation activities does my client enjoy that might facilitate mastery and generalization of targeted relaxation?*
4. **Technique preferences.** *Which specific techniques, or technique components, does my client prefer?*
5. **R-State experiences and preferences.** *Which R-States does my client experience? Which R-States does my client desire? Which techniques, or technique components, appear to facilitate these R-States.*
6. **R-Attitudes.** *What R-Attitudes does my client appear to display? How might we modify these?*
7. **R-Beliefs.** *What R-Beliefs does my client display? How might these be incorporated into relaxation?*
8. **Problems and logistics.** *What problems or difficulties is my client experiencing with relaxation? How might training be modified to take these into account?*

TABLE 2.1   Script for Grand Tour Lecture

In this workshop we will look at one of the most powerful and popular tools for therapy and self-improvement—relaxation. Relaxation has many uses—managing stress and pain, treating insomnia, enhancing health, increasing work productivity and sports performance. And relaxation is used in just about every helping profession—psychology, medicine, nursing, counseling, sports, and many others.

Today we are going to look at a new approach, called ABC relaxation. There are many approaches to relaxation—yoga, imagery, and meditation are just a few. How is ABC Relaxation different? To understand, we need to take a look at history. For thousands of years, relaxation techniques have been handed down by experts. A wise person, psychologist, or doctor invents a new technique and teaches it to followers. This is the top down approach to relaxation.

[PUT ON BOARD]

RELAXATION EXPERT

↓

IDEAS ABOUT RELAXATION

Researchers at Chicago's Roosevelt University Stress Institute have been looking at relaxation differently, by asking doers rather than the teachers—from the ground up, not the top down, like this:

IDEAS ABOUT RELAXATION

↑

THOUSANDS OF ACTUAL REAL-LIFE PRACTITIONERS OF
EVERY FORM OF RELAXATION

This may seem like an obvious thing to do. Relaxation techniques have been around for 5,000 years. The reason no one has ever done this before is that we haven't had the computer power. For the first time in history, technology has sufficiently advanced so that we can ask this type of important question. And the answers are sur-

(continued)

TABLE 2.1   *(continued)*

prising. In this workshop I would like to share with you some recent discoveries about relaxation.

Ten years ago, scientists at the Roosevelt University Stress Institute began the largest and longest scientific investigation ever conducted on relaxation. This "Large Scale Relaxation Project" involved over 6,000 participants—people from all cultures and religions. The researchers looked at just about every type of relaxation you can think of, breathing exercises, muscle relaxation, yoga stretching, visualization, meditation, prayer, and even everyday relaxation activities like pleasure reading, listening to music, watching TV, taking walks, and even petting pets and humming.

The coordinator of this research effort, Dr. Jonathan Smith, summarizes the goal of this massive project this way:

"We decided to look not at the wisdom of a single person, but the collective wisdom of a thousand voices."

And here is what the researchers found. Put simply, for decades the relaxation exerts have been wrong. Let me explain. For years the "top down" relaxation world view has been this:

> All approaches to relaxation are the same and have the same effect—
> reduced body tension. It doesn't matter what type of relaxation you
> practice, because they all have the same effect—reduced body tension.

In fact, different approaches to relaxation have different effects for different people. One size doesn't fit all. What works for you may not work for your neighbor. But the most remarkable discovery was just what the effect of relaxation really is. Once again, it is not what the experts were saying—and continue to say.

All approaches to relaxation evoke a fundamental process of healing and growth in which one withdraws from the efforts of the day, recovers, and opens up to the world. Dr. Smith has termed this the Cycle of Renewal. The idea of a cyclical renewal process has been around for several millennia and can be manifest at many levels. World religions speak of global cycles of death and rebirth, repentance and forgiveness, as well as acceptance and enlightenment. Professional approaches to relaxation involve mastering the discipline of withdrawing from everyday stress for healing and recovery, and returning to the world refreshed and restored. And each time we pause and sigh we display a moment of relaxation and renewal.

Relaxation States

Researchers have identified what might be called the "secret of the Cycle of Renewal." We know the Cycle of Renewal is working

TABLE 2.1 *(continued)*

in relaxation when we experience a set of powerful psychological relaxation states, called R-States. R-States are what actually contribute to the effectiveness of relaxation. They are part of the inner workings of the Cycle of Renewal. Here are the R-States that have been identified so far.

[PUT ON BOARD]

Relaxation States (R-States)

1: Sleepiness
2: Disengagement
3: Physical Relaxation
4: Mental Quiet
5: Mental Relaxation
6: Strength and Awareness
7: Joy and Happiness
8: Love and Thankfulness
9: Prayerfulness

These nine R-States are the key to relaxation's promise for enhancing health, well-being, and productivity. R-States make all of relaxation, from massage to meditation, work. If an approach does not evoke an R-State, it will not work.

Let's take a look at each R-State. R-States 1 and 2, Sleepiness and Disengagement, involve pulling away from the cares and concerns of the world. One takes a "mental vacation," often feeling "detached, far away, and distant." Physical Relaxation is an absence of body tension. Mental Quiet is a thought-free state of inner quiet. Mental Relaxation is a state of peace and inner ease, free of stress and conflict. Once we have recovered from the toxic effects of the pressures of the world, we experience the R-States Strength and Awareness, Joy, and Love and Thankfulness. And eventually, if we continue relaxing with sustained awareness, putting aside our personal cares, concerns, and even feelings of pleasure and joy, we can begin to see glimpses of a deeper universe that underlies everything. We experience reverence and Prayerfulness.

The notion of R-States makes more sense if we take a look at an example.

Joan is an accountant. She works long and hard, and lives under high levels of chronic stress—client deadlines, complex reports, budgets, returning phone calls, and so on. One day Joan decides to take a week off, and ride her bike into a nearby

(continued)

TABLE 2.1 *(continued)*

mountain retreat. The night before, she had retired to bed and experiences the first R-State *Sleepiness*. The next day, she packs her gear, gets on her bike, and begins to ride down the street to a nearby path. After about half an hour, Joan reaches a wooded park. She looks back and sees her home town in the distance. She sighs, very glad that her home and hectic work are beginning to feel like far away memories. She experiences the R-State *Disengagement*.

After a day of riding, Joan reaches a camping spot. She puts her bike away and sits on a soft patch of grass. She stretches, lies down, and closes her eyes. She has a nice sensation of "sinking in" the soft grass. Her body feels limp, warm, and heavy. Joan feels *Physical Relaxation*. In a few minutes, Joan notices that her mind is still without thought. She experiences *Mental Quiet*. After about fifteen minutes, Joan begins to notice how calm and peaceful her mind feels. She is now truly at ease, safe from the world of conflict and confrontation. This is *Mental Relaxation*. Free from her conflicts at work and home, Joan opens her eyes, notices how refreshed and renewed she feels. She is focused and clear. This is *Strength and Awareness*. The pressures of the day a distant memory, the body relaxed, and the mind calm and clear, she can begin to see clearly the sky above and the trees around. She is struck with their beauty and wonder. She feels a sense of deep harmony with the world. She feels *Joy*. Joan enjoys this beautiful feeling a few minutes, feeling the R-State *Love and Thankfulness*, grateful that she has had the opportunity to experience this special moment, wishing her friends were there to share it with her. Evening approaches. The air is quiet. Joan gazes at the sky above and sees the emergence with the first evening star in the vast heavens. And for an instant Joan is struck with a sense of awe and wonder of the deep world around. Joan experiences a moment of *Prayerfulness*.

Relaxation researchers have made a second discovery. The benefits of relaxation are not automatic, but depend on what you believe. Eight relaxation beliefs, *R-Beliefs* enhance and deepen the R-States one can experience.

Relaxation Beliefs (R-Beliefs)

1: Deeper Perspective
   (Put your concerns in deeper perspective)

TABLE 2.1 *(continued)*

2: God
   (Trust God's love and guidance)
3: Inner Wisdom
   (Trust the healing wisdom of the body)
4: Love
   (Relate to others with love & compassion)
5: Honesty
   (Be honest, open with yourself and others)
6: Acceptance
   (Accept things than can't be changed)
7: Taking It Easy
   (Know when to let go and take it easy)
8: Optimism
   (View your hassles with optimism)

Of these, research suggests that three beliefs may be the most powerful: belief in inner wisdom, acceptance, and optimism.

It is important to recognize that R-Beliefs are different from coping beliefs. R-Beliefs help one relax; coping beliefs (like "plan ahead," "consider the consequences of your actions") help one deal with the hassles of active living.

The Inner Secrets of Relaxation

I would now like to share with you the secret of relaxation. What is relaxation? The top down approach offers many partial and conflicting answers. However, if we put aside the claims of experts and tradition, and look at what practitioners of diverse relaxation traditions do, we see a common thread. All approaches to relaxation involve the act of sustaining passive simple focus. This is the act that makes relaxation work. But what does this mean? How is this different from what we ordinarily do?

First, everyday life is *effortful*. We plan and strive to achieve our daily goals, anticipate the future, and reflect upon the past. Furthermore, life is moving and changing, it is *discursive* (from the Latin "cursere" for "moving to and fro"). We plan schedules, vacations, and shopping lists; even in idle moments of fantasy, our thoughts ramble from image to image. Discursive effort is good; indeed, it is the very key to success. If you go shopping, you plan which store to go to, how to get there, what to buy, how to pay, and how to get your purchase home. For every single thing you do in life, if you want to succeed or get ahead, you must exert at least some discursive planning effort.

(continued)

TABLE 2.1 *(continued)*

There is one exception. The key to all forms of relaxation is sustained passive simple focus the opposite of what we usually do to succeed. At first this might seem like a simple thing to do. Everyone has experienced special moments of simple letting go and focusing. Perhaps you were gazing at a sunset, and for an instant golden rays burst through violet clouds. Briefly, you felt deep peace and beauty. Or you may have encountered the secret of simply letting go and simply focusing in relaxing music. Moments of simply focusing and simply letting go are part of life's treasures; but such moments come and go quickly. The sun sets. The music ends. We go on with our day's work. The secret of relaxation is to sustain the moment. This is a very difficult thing to do, something like balancing a basketball on a calm and steady fingertip. Special relaxation techniques, like imagery, yoga, breathing exercises, and meditation, help.

The ABC Relaxation Method

Relaxation techniques are not self-hypnosis or religious ritual. They are respected professional tools perfected through decades of careful scientific research and used by psychologists and counselors around the world. Relaxation can be very powerful. It can help us resist and recover from illness. It can enhance creativity and productivity. It can be an important part of effective stress management.

The ABC Relaxation Method offers a new way of exploring a timeless discipline. The top down approach says one size fits all. It doesn't matter what relaxation technique you learn because they all work the same. We have seen that this idea is clearly wrong. Different techniques have different effects and work for different people. The ABC method of relaxation makes use of this discovery. It has three steps.

1. *Preliminary training.* Begin by learning, not one, but five approaches to relaxation (PMR, AT, breathing exercises, yoga stretching, imagery, and meditation). Make sure to learn "purified" versions of each approach, so you can identify the unique relaxation effects of each.
2. *Exercise selection.* Select which specific exercises seem to work best.
3. *Program development.* Fashion exercises, words suggestive of desired relaxation states (R-States), and affirmations of relaxation-supportive beliefs (R-Beliefs) into a per-

---

TABLE 2.1 *(continued)*

---

sonal practice program that has both clinical and aesthetic integrity.

A Closing Image

What is the goal of relaxation? You may learn relaxation for a specific, limited goal, for example, treating a headache or insomnia. This is perfectly fine. But there is more to relaxation than symptom relief. The special act of sustaining passive simple focus can open new doors of understanding. Let me close with something of a parable, an image taken from modern astronomy. It is an image that also conveys very nicely the promise of relaxation.

One of the most important events in space science has been the launching of the Hubble telescope. Ten times more powerful than any telescope on earth, the orbiting Hubble can see where no one has seen before. Two things make the Hubble an especially powerful tool. First, it can examine the heavens undistracted by the city lights, haze, and noise of earth. It is above all of that. Second, the Hubble can sustain its focus, unmoved, for hours, days, and even weeks. No earth telescope can do this—shifting continents, passing traffic, changes in the atmosphere, and the rotation of the planet itself mean that the gaze of any land-based telescope is never perfectly steady.

For 10 days in late 1995, astronomers conducted an experiment that changed our vision of the universe. It was a study that had never, and indeed could never have been conducted before. In the "deep field experiment," astronomers aimed the Hubble toward a patch of space that has always appeared completely empty, a small dark spot of sky where earth telescopes indicated nothing existed. (For star gazers, this empty area is close to the handle of the "Big Dipper," and is about one hundredth the size of the moon.) What really exists in this empty space? After a full two weeks of sustained, unmoving, focus, the Hubble had a surprising answer—one trillion stars extending to the very edge of the universe. Thousands of galaxies. Each containing billions of stars. Astronomers have concluded that this discovery transforms our vision of the Universe. It is far richer than anyone ever imagined. The deep field experiment shows that what we thought was empty space is filled with an unimaginable richness of stars. And the key to this discovery was sustained passive simple focus. This, as we have seen, is also the key to relaxation.

TABLE 2.2   Script for Grand Tour Experiential Workshop

PART 1: EXPLANATION AND RATIONALE

In this workshop we will look at one of the most powerful and popular tools for therapy and self-improvement—relaxation. Relaxation has many uses—managing stress and pain, treating insomnia, enhancing health, increasing work productivity and sports performance. And relaxation is used in just about every helping profession—psychology, medicine, nursing, counseling, sports, and many others.

Today we are going to look at a new approach, called ABC Relaxation. There are many approaches to relaxation—yoga, imagery, and meditation are just a few. How is ABC Relaxation different? To understand, we need to take a look at history. For thousands of years, relaxation techniques have been handed down by experts. A wise person, psychologist, or doctor invents a new technique and teaches it to followers. This is the top down approach to relaxation.

[PUT ON BOARD]

RELAXATION EXPERT

↓

IDEAS ABOUT RELAXATION

Researchers at Chicago's Roosevelt University Stress Institute have looking at relaxation differently, by asking doers rather than the teachers—from the ground up, not the top down, like this:

IDEAS ABOUT RELAXATION

↑

THOUSANDS OF ACTUAL REAL-LIFE PRACTITIONERS OF
EVERY FORM OF RELAXATION

This may seem like an obvious thing to do. Relaxation techniques have been around for 5,000 years. The reason no one has ever done this before is we haven't had the computer power. For the first time in history, technology has sufficiently advanced so that we can ask this type of important question.

TABLE 2.2 *(continued)*

And the answers are surprising. In this workshop I would like to share with you some recent discoveries about relaxation, and then demonstrate how you can make these same discoveries yourself with a new approach to relaxation.

Ten years ago, scientists at the Roosevelt University Stress Institute began the largest and longest scientific investigation ever conducted on relaxation. This "Large Scale Relaxation Project, " involved over 6,000 participants—people from all cultures and religions. The researchers looked at just about every type of relaxation you can think of, breathing exercises, muscle relaxation, yoga stretching, visualization, meditation, prayer, and even everyday relaxation activities like pleasure reading, listening to music, watching TV, taking walks, and even petting pets and humming.

The coordinator of this research effort, Dr. Jonathan Smith, summarizes the goal of this massive 10-year project this way: "We decided to look not at the wisdom of a single person, but the collective wisdom of a thousand voices."

And researchers found that for fifty years the relaxation experts have been wrong. Let me explain. For years the "top down" relaxation world view has been this:

All approaches to relaxation are the same and have the same effect—reduced body tension. It doesn't matter what type of relaxation you practice, because they all have the same effect—reduced body tension.

In fact, different approaches to relaxation have different effects for different people. One size doesn't fit all. What works for you may not work for your neighbor. But the most remarkable discovery was just what the effect of relaxation really is. Once again, it is not what the experts were saying—and continue to say.

All approaches to relaxation evoke a fundamental process of healing and growth in which one withdraws from the efforts of the day, recovers, and opens up to the world. Dr. Smith has termed this the Cycle of Renewal. The idea of a cyclical renewal process has been around for several millennia and can be manifest at many levels. World religions speak of global cycles of death and rebirth, repentance and forgiveness, as well as acceptance and enlightenment. Professional approaches to relaxation involve mastering the discipline of withdrawing from everyday stress for healing and recovery, and returning to the world refreshed and restored. And each time we pause and sigh we display a moment of relaxation and renewal.

Researchers have identified what might be called the "secret of the Cycle of Renewal." We know the Cycle of Renewal is working

(continued)

TABLE 2.2 *(continued)*

in relaxation when we experience a set of powerful psychological relaxation states, called R-States. R-States are what actually contribute to the effectiveness of relaxation. They are part of the inner workings of the Cycle of Renewal. Here are the R-States that have been identified so far.

[PUT THE R-STATES ON THE BOARD, AS NAMED]
1. Sleepiness
2. Disengagement
3. Physical Relaxation
4. Mental Quiet
5. Mental Relaxation
6. Strength and Awareness
7. Joy
8. Love and Thankfulness
9. Prayerfulness

Let's take a look at the world of R-States. Some R-States are easy to recognize and involve pulling away from a stressful world and recovering from it: for example—Sleepiness, feeling Physically Relaxed and limp, feeling Mentally Relaxed and at peace. Another R-State, Mental Quiet, is a little unfamiliar to many people. This is a special state in which the mind is completely calm and quiet, silent without any thoughts. Another R-State may also seem a little unfamiliar—feeling far away from the cares of the world, indifferent, and detached. This state is called Disengagement.

Once tensions are calmed, and we have recovered from a day's wear and tear, we may experience higher R-States that involve opening up to the world. Things may seem clearer and we experience the R-State Strength and Awareness. Once Strengthened and Aware, we can begin to see the wonders of the world around us; we may feel such R-States as Joy, Love and Thankfulness, and even, in special deep moments, Prayerful reverence.

But these R-States may seem a little dry. So let me tell you a simple story that illustrates the notion of R-States and may make them more meaningful to you.

> Joan is an accountant. She works long and hard, and lives under high levels of chronic stress—client deadlines, complex reports, budgets, returning phone calls, and so on. Joan decides to take a week off, and ride her bike into a nearby mountain retreat. The night before, she has retired to bed and experiences the first R-State, *Sleepiness*. The next day, she packs her gear, gets on her bike, and begins to ride down the street to a nearby path. After about half an hour, Joan reaches a

TABLE 2.2 *(continued)*

wooded park. She looks back, and sees her home town in the distance. She sighs, very glad that her home, and hectic work, are beginning to feel like far away memories. She experiences the R-State *Disengagement*.

After a day of riding, Joan reaches a camping spot. She puts her bike away and sits on a soft patch of grass. She stretches, lies down, and closes her eyes. Her mind is still, without thought. She experiences *Mental Quiet*. Her body feels wonderfully relaxed, "loose and limp." She has a nice sensation of "sinking in" the soft grass. Joan feels *Physical Relaxation*. After about fifteen minutes, Joan begins to notice how calm and peaceful her mind feels. She is now truly at ease, safe from the world of conflict and confrontation. This is *Mental Relaxation*. Free from her conflicts at work and home, Joan opens her eyes, notices how refreshed and renewed she feels. She is focused and clear. This is *Strength and Awareness*. The pressures of the day a distant memory, the body relaxed, and the mind calm and clear, she can begin to see clearly the sky above and the trees around. She is struck with their beauty and wonder. She feels a sense of deep harmony with the world. She feels *Joy*. Joan enjoys this beautiful feeling a few minutes, feeling the R-State *Love and Thankfulness*, grateful that she has had the opportunity to experience this special moment, wishing her friends were there to share it with her. Evening approaches. The air is quiet. Joan gazes at the sky above and sees the emergence with the first evening star in the vast heavens. And for an instant Joan is struck with a sense of awe and wonder of the deep world around. Joan experiences a moment of *Prayerfulness*.

Joan discovered all nine R-States. Each is powerful in and of itself. You may not experience them together, like Joan did.

We can now underline the importance of this discovery. It is not an idea handed down by an expert in one technique, or an idea from a single book. The notion of R-States is truly a common insight, the universal voice of wisdom rising from thousands of practitioners of all types of relaxation.

Dr. Smith proposes that R-States are what make relaxation work. No matter how much you pay your relaxation therapist, unless their technique evokes at least some R-States, you are wasting your money. No matter how many years you spend in yoga or meditation class, unless you discover at least some R-States, you are wasting your money. No matter how fervently you desire or pray for relaxation to lead to health and well being, unless you can experience

(continued)

TABLE 2.2   *(continued)*
R-States in relaxation, your thoughts and desires will remain wishful thinking.

We can put this theory on the board:

[PUT ON BOARD]

RELAXATION TECHNIQUE

↓

R-STATES

↓

HEALING, PRODUCTIVITY, WELL-BEING

Professional relaxation techniques are not self-hypnosis or religious ritual. They are respected professional tools perfected through decades of careful scientific research and used by psychologists and counselors around the world. Relaxation can be very powerful. It can help us resist and recover from illness. It can enhance creativity and productivity. It can be an important part of effective stress management.

Here are the relaxation techniques used most often by professionals:

- Professional Muscle Relaxation (or "Progressive Muscle Relaxation")
- Self-Suggestion (or "Autogenic Training")
- Breathing Exercises
- Yoga Stretching
- Visualization, Imagery, and Prayer
- Meditation

PUT TECHNIQUES ON BOARD, NEXT TO R-STATES:

	Muscle Relaxation Autogenics	Stretching Breathing	Imagery	Meditation
Sleep	_____	_____	_____	_____
Disengagement	_____	_____	_____	_____
Physical Relaxation	_____	_____	_____	_____
Mental Quiet	_____	_____	_____	_____

TABLE 2.2 *(continued)*

Mental Relaxation	____	____	____	____
Strength and Awareness	____	____	____	____
Joy	____	____	____	____
Love and Thankfulness	____	____	____	____
Prayerfulness	____	____	____	____

Some of these you may have heard of, some not. Some you may have positive thoughts about, some negative. You may even be a practitioner of a technique and think it is better than all others. Whatever you think about these techniques, please keep an open mind and remember that relaxation as taught by licensed psychologists can be quite different from the phony hyped up fads you read about and see on TV.

In a minute we will sample the major approaches to relaxation used by professionals. We will ask this simple question. Do they all have the same effect, as believed by many? Or do different techniques have different effects? [FOR TAPE: On the other side of this tape, you will have a chance to try these techniques and decide for yourself. You can now remove this tape, turn it over, and relax to the worlds of relaxation.]

So it is now time to take a break from the hectic pace of everyday and enjoy ourselves. From time to time, I will ask you how you feel. For example, I may ask "do you feel at ease and at peace?" If you feel this, raise your index finger, like this [DEMONSTRATE]. I will take a tally of how many people experience this and put it on the board. This way, at the end of the workshop we can see what R-States were experienced for each technique.

Finally, I need to assure you that what we will be doing is not hypnosis. You will be in charge. All you have to do is enjoy each exercise as I present the instructions. And what we will be doing is not religion. Although the exercises can and have been a part of religion, they are tools valid in and of themselves. Books, music, and art are used in religion; and they are valid forms of expression in themselves.

I also need to warn you that what we will be doing is a learning experience designed to introduce you to the types of relaxation treatments available. Our workshop is not a treatment for any disorder, or any type of psychotherapy, counseling, or stress manage-

(continued)

TABLE 2.2 *(continued)*

---

ment. It is simply too brief to have any lasting therapeutic effect. When used in actual therapeutic treatment, relaxation training must take weeks and months with daily practice. And it must be taught by a qualified clinical psychologist or licensed mental health professional.

PART 2: EXERCISE DEMONSTRATION

We are going to take a relaxing vacation. Over the next 20 minutes or so we will sample the most widely used approaches to professional relaxation. You will have a chance to answer for yourself the important question: Are all approaches to relaxation alike, as many professionals think? Or do they have different effects?

Let's begin. Please make sure you are sitting in a comfortable position. Rest your feet comfortably on the floor. It is OK to let go and slump over a little. Let your head bow a little as you relax. And close your eyes.

Let go of the cares and concerns of the day. This is your time to enjoy the different worlds of relaxation.

Progressive Muscle Relaxation (Overt) and Autogenic Training

Let's begin by attending to our shoulder muscles. While keeping the rest of your body loose and relaxed, shrug your shoulders *now*. Create a nice, good squeeze. Feel it throughout your shoulder muscles.

Now let go. Let yourself go completely limp.

[PAUSE]

Let the tension begin to dissolve and flow away.

[PAUSE]

Begin to sink into a pleasant state of relaxation.

[PAUSE]

Let yourself become more and more relaxed.

[PAUSE]

Let's try that once again. Focus your attention on your

TABLE 2.2 *(continued)*

shoulder muscles. And shrug them *now*. Create a nice, good shrug. Feel the tension as it squeezes out of your shoulders.

And let go. Go completely limp.

[PAUSE]

Let the tension begin to flow away.

[PAUSE]

Your muscles begin to feel more limp and loose as the tension flows away.

[PAUSE]

Let yourself sink deeper and deeper into relaxation.

[PAUSE]

Very good. Let's try another exercise that is very similar.

Focus on the muscles at the back of your neck. Slowly tilt your head back, and easily squeeze the muscles. Do this now. Let the tension grow. Feel a nice, complete squeeze.

And let go. Let your muscles go completely limp.

[PAUSE]

Let the tension dissolve and begin to flow away.

[PAUSE]

The muscles may begin to tingle as tension is released.

[PAUSE]

Let yourself sink deeper and deeper into relaxation

[PAUSE]

And let's try that again. Slowly tilt your head back, and easily squeeze the muscles.

Let the tension grow. Feel a nice, complete squeeze.

And let go. Let your muscles go completely limp.

[PAUSE]

Let the tension dissolve and begin to flow away.

[PAUSE]

The muscles may begin to tingle as tension is released.

[PAUSE]

(continued)

TABLE 2.2   *(continued)*

Let yourself sink deeper and deeper into relaxation.

[PAUSE]

There, that was very good.

[PAUSE]

And now focus on both arms.

[PAUSE]

Tighten up both arms, by bending at the elbow, trying to touch your fist and your shoulder, like this. Tighten both arms now.

[PAUSE]

Let the tension grow.

[PAUSE]

Feel the tension.

[PAUSE]

And go limp, resting your arms in your lap.

[PAUSE]

Let yourself go.

[PAUSE]

Let the tensions begin to dissolve and flow away.

[PAUSE]

Sink deeper and deeper into pleasant relaxation.

[PAUSE]

Far away from the cares of the day.

[PAUSE]

And once again, tense up both arms now.

[PAUSE]

Let the tension grow.

[PAUSE]

Feel the squeeze.

[PAUSE]

TABLE 2.2 *(continued)*

And go limp.

[PAUSE]

Let the tension flow out.

[PAUSE]

Let yourself become more and more loose and limp.

[PAUSE]

Let yourself become more completely relaxed.

[PAUSE]

Let yourself continue to sink deeper and deeper into relaxation.

Far away from the cares and concerns of the day.

There is nothing you have to do.

And quietly attend to your hands.

Let the words, "warm and heavy" float through your mind, like an echo.

[PAUSE]

Warm and heavy.

[PAUSE]

Warm and heavy.

[PAUSE]

Let these words simply float over and over, at a very slow and lazy pace.

[PAUSE]

There is nothing you have to do.

[PAUSE]

Hands and arms warm and heavy.

[PAUSE]

Like you are resting in warm sand on the beach.

[PAUSE]

Warm and heavy.

[PAUSE]

So warm and heavy as they relax more and more.

(continued)

TABLE 2.2   *(continued)*

[PAUSE]

Warm and heavy, like they are sinking in warm and heavy sand.

[PAUSE]

Let the tensions slowly melt away. Warm and heavy.

[PAUSE]

Let yourself sink into a deep state of relaxation.

[PAUSE]

Hands and arms, warm and heavy.

[PAUSE]

There is nothing for you to do.

[PAUSE]

Here, nothing matters.

[PAUSE]

Like warm sun melting the tensions away.

[PAUSE]

Warm and heavy. Warm and heavy.

[PAUSE]

You are far away from the pressures and cares of the world.

[PAUSE]

Let the tensions begin to flow away.

[PAUSE 10 SECONDS]

How did these exercises make you feel?

With your eyes closed, ask yourself, how do you feel right now?

If you feel drowsy or sleepy, please raise your right index finger. [RECORD ON BOARD NUMBER OF RESPONSES BY "SLEEPINESS"]

If you feel distant, far away, or detached, raise your finger. [RECORD ON BOARD BY "DISENGAGEMENT"]

If your body feels physically relaxed, loose and limp, maybe your muscles feeling warm and heavy, raise your finger [RECORD BY "PHYSICAL RELAXATION"]

If your mind is quiet, silent, without thought, raise your finger. [RECORD BY "MENTAL QUIET"]

TABLE 2.2 *(continued)*

If you feel at ease, at peace, and maybe contented, raise your finger [RECORD BY "MENTAL RELAXATION"]

Do you feel aware, focused, strengthened, or energized? [RECORD BY "STRENGTH AND AWARENESS"]

Do you feel happy or joyful? [RECORD BY "JOY"]

Do you feel loving or thankful? [RECORD BY "LOVE AND THANKFULNESS"]

Do you feel Prayerful, reverent, or spiritual? [RECORD BY "PRAYERFUL"]

And now we continue.

We will now continue our tour of relaxation by trying a different set of exercises.

This time, sit up straight in a comfortable and alert position. Make sure your feet are flat on the floor. And close your eyes.

The exercises we are about to try may help you feel relaxed and refreshed. With a clear and peaceful mind, we will let ourselves become open to and enjoy interesting new worlds of relaxation.

Yoga Stretching and Breathing Exercises

Begin by letting both arms hang to your sides.

[PAUSE]

Focus on your right hand and arm.

Slowly, smoothly, and gently, begin to lift your right arm from your side, like the hand of a clock or the wing of a bird.

[PAUSE]

Very slowly, smoothly, and gently, as if you were balancing a feather on your hand.

[PAUSE. CONTINUE IN PACE WITH CLIENT.]

Very easily, lift your arm higher and higher.

[PAUSE. CONTINUE IN PACE WITH CLIENT.]

Take your time. Very smooth and gentle. Tracing a circle in the air.

[PAUSE, CONTINUE IN PACE WITH CLIENT.]

(continued)

TABLE 2.2 *(continued)*

Lift your arm and hand over your head and reach to the sky, all the way.

[PAUSE. CONTINUE IN PACE WITH CLIENT.]

Feel the good stretch all along your arm and hand. And reach over your head, pointing to the left. Stretch every inch of your arm and hand.

[PAUSE. CONTINUE IN PACE WITH CLIENT.]

And, when you are ready, gently unstretch. Very slowly, smoothly, and gently, return your arm, like the hand of a clock.

[PAUSE. CONTINUE IN PACE WITH CLIENT.]

And when you are ready, let your arm and hand hang to your side.

[PAUSE, WAIT FOR CLIENT TO FINISH]

And once again, slowly, smoothly, and gently, begin to lift your right arm from your side, like the hand of a clock or the wing of a bird.

[PAUSE]

Very slowly, smoothly, and gently, as if you were balancing a feather on your hand.

[PAUSE. CONTINUE IN PACE WITH CLIENT.]

Very easily, lift your arm higher and higher.

[PAUSE. CONTINUE IN PACE WITH CLIENT.]

Take your time. Very smooth and gentle. Tracing a circle in the air.

[PAUSE, CONTINUE IN PACE WITH CLIENT.]

Lift your arm and hand over your head and reach to the sky, all the way.

[PAUSE. CONTINUE IN PACE WITH CLIENT.]

Feel the good stretch all along your arm and hand. And reach over your head, pointing to the left. Stretch every inch of your arm and hand.

[PAUSE. CONTINUE IN PACE WITH CLIENT.]

And, when you are ready, gently unstretch. Very slowly, smoothly, and gently, return your arm, like the hand of a clock.

[PAUSE. CONTINUE IN PACE WITH CLIENT.]

TABLE 2.2 *(continued)*

And when you are ready, let your arm and hand hang to your side.

[PAUSE. CONTINUE IN PACE WITH CLIENT.]

Very good. Now, let's try that with the other hand and arm.

Slowly, smoothly, and gently, begin to lift them up.

[PAUSE. CONTINUE IN PACE WITH CLIENT.]

Higher and higher, like the hand of a clock, or the wing of a bird. Very smoothly and gently.

[PAUSE. CONTINUE IN PACE WITH CLIENT.]

Take your time. There is no reason to hurry.

[PAUSE. CONTINUE IN PACE WITH CLIENT.]

Create a nice good stretch all the way.

[PAUSE. CONTINUE IN PACE WITH CLIENT.]

Point to the sky, higher and higher. Feel the stretch. And, when you are ready, reach and point to the other side.

[PAUSE. CONTINUE IN PACE WITH CLIENT.]

Create a nice good stretch.

[PAUSE. CONTINUE IN PACE WITH CLIENT.]

Gently unstretch, and very slowly, return your hand to your lap.

[PAUSE. WAIT FOR CLIENT TO FINISH]

And again, Slowly, smoothly, and gently, begin to lift them up.

[PAUSE. CONTINUE IN PACE WITH CLIENT.]

Higher and higher, like the hand of a clock, or the wing of a bird. Very smoothly and gently.

[PAUSE. CONTINUE IN PACE WITH CLIENT.]

Take your time. There is no reason to hurry.

[PAUSE. CONTINUE IN PACE WITH CLIENT.]

Create a nice good stretch all the way.

[PAUSE. CONTINUE IN PACE WITH CLIENT.]

Point to the sky, higher and higher. Feel the stretch. And, when you are ready, reach and point to the other side.

[PAUSE. CONTINUE IN PACE WITH CLIENT.]

Create a nice good stretch.

(continued)

TABLE 2.2   *(continued)*

[PAUSE. CONTINUE IN PACE WITH CLIENT.]

Gently unstretch, and very slowly, return your hands to your lap.

[PAUSE. CONTINUE IN PACE WITH CLIENT.]

Take your time. Very slowly and gently.

[PAUSE. CONTINUE IN PACE WITH CLIENT.]

We are now going to bow, and stretch.

[PAUSE]

Let both harms hang to your sides.

[PAUSE]

And slowly begin to bow forward.

[PAUSE. CONTINUE IN PACE WITH CLIENT.]

Do not force yourself down.

[PAUSE. CONTINUE IN PACE WITH CLIENT.]

Let gravity pull your torso down on its own.

[PAUSE. CONTINUE IN PACE WITH CLIENT.]

All you have to do is feel the gentle stretch along your back.

[PAUSE. CONTINUE IN PACE WITH CLIENT.]

Very smoothly and gently.

[PAUSE. CONTINUE IN PACE WITH CLIENT.]

You can take a little breath whenever you wish.

[PAUSE. CONTINUE IN PACE WITH CLIENT.]

Bow further and further

[PAUSE. CONTINUE IN PACE WITH CLIENT.]

Feel a good stretch all along your body.

[PAUSE. CONTINUE IN PACE WITH CLIENT.]

As you stretch completely.

[PAUSE. CONTINUE IN PACE WITH CLIENT.]

And, when you are ready, slowly, smoothly, and gently unstretch.

[PAUSE. CONTINUE IN PACE WITH CLIENT.]

TABLE 2.2 *(continued)*

Slowly, smoothly, and gently raise your arms to the sky.

[PAUSE. CONTINUE IN PACE WITH CLIENT.]

Stretch higher and higher.

[PAUSE. CONTINUE IN PACE WITH CLIENT.]

Feel a good full and comfortable stretch.

[PAUSE. CONTINUE IN PACE WITH CLIENT.]

Stretch and arch your back.

[PAUSE. CONTINUE IN PACE WITH CLIENT.]

And, when you are ready, slowly, smoothly, and gently unstretch.

And attend to your breathing.

[PAUSE]

Attend to how you are breathing.

[PAUSE]

Let yourself breathe easily and naturally. Very smoothly and gently.

[PAUSE]

And now, take a full deep breath. Very smooth and even. Filling your lungs with refreshing air. And pause.

And when you are ready, slowly let the air flow out through your lips, as if you were blowing on a candle, just enough to make the flame flicker.

[PAUSE. CONTINUE IN PACE WITH CLIENT.]

And continue to breathe at a normal, relaxed pace. There is no reason to force yourself to breathe in any particular way. Just breathe easily and naturally.

[PAUSE 15 SECONDS]

And, just like before, take a slow, full breath. Very easily, fill your lungs all the way.

[PAUSE. CONTINUE IN PACE WITH CLIENT.]

When you are ready, slowly and gently exhale through your lips, as before.

(continued)

TABLE 2.2 *(continued)*

[PAUSE. CONTINUE IN PACE WITH CLIENT.]

And continue to breathe naturally.

How did these exercises make you feel?

With your eyes closed, ask yourself, how do you feel right now?

If you feel drowsy or sleepy, please raise your right index finger. [RECORD ON BOARD NUMBER OF RESPONSES BY "SLEEPINESS"]

If you feel distant, far away, or detached, raise your finger. [RECORD ON BOARD BY "DISENGAGEMENT"]

If your body feels physically relaxed, loose and limp, maybe your muscles feeling warm and heavy, raise your finger [RECORD BY "PHYSICAL RELAXATION"]

If your mind is quiet, silent, without thought, raise your finger. [RECORD BY "MENTAL QUIET"]

If you feel at ease, at peace, and maybe contented, raise your finger [RECORD BY "MENTAL RELAXATION"]

Do you feel aware, focused, strengthened, or energized? [RECORD BY "STRENGTH AND AWARENESS"]

Do you feel happy or joyful? [RECORD BY "JOY"]

Do you feel loving or thankful? [RECORD BY "LOVE AND THANKFULNESS"]

Do you feel Prayerful, reverent, or spiritual? [RECORD BY "PRAYERFUL"]

And now we continue.

Imagery

Gently let go of what you are attending to.

With your eyes closed, think of a very peaceful and relaxing outdoor setting.

[PAUSE]

Perhaps this is a favorite vacation spot, or a distant relaxing destination of your dreams.

[PAUSE 10 SECONDS]

Think of a relaxing setting.

TABLE 2.2 *(continued)*

And imagine you are there.

[PAUSE]

Enjoy it with all your senses.

[PAUSE]

What do you see?

[PAUSE]

Perhaps you can see the clear peaceful sky. Maybe a soft and relaxing cloud or two.

[PAUSE]

Perhaps there are beautiful green trees, grass, or flowers.

[PAUSE]

Maybe you can see a wonderful pond, river, or lake.

[PAUSE]

What relaxing sounds do you hear?

[PAUSE]

Perhaps you hear an occasional dove singing overhead.

Or the sound of the wind in the grass and trees.

Or water splashing in a nearby brook or pond.

[PAUSE]

You may feel the refreshing touch of air and sun on your skin. Cooling. Warm. Refreshing.

[PAUSE]

What relaxing fragrances can you notice?

Perhaps you can smell the clean, fresh waters and trees.

[PAUSE]

Take a few seconds to enjoy this pleasant setting. Let yourself enjoy it with all yours Senses, and notice what you see, hear, feel, and smell.

[PAUSE 20 SECONDS]

[OPTIONAL SUPPLEMENT]

(continued)

TABLE 2.2 *(continued)*

And now in your mind's eye begin to look around.

[PAUSE]

In the distance is a cabin.

The cabin is warm and friendly.

[PAUSE]

And far away you notice a person taking a peaceful stroll.

[PAUSE]

This place has a message of peace and wonder for you.

Perhaps it is just the good feeling of being there.

Or perhaps a special message, one just for you, appears.

[PAUSE]

There are two ways this message may appear.

In the cabin, one door is partly open. If you open the door all the way you may find a message.

Or the person in the distance slowly walks closer to you.

You recognize this person as someone very wise and good, a teacher, relative, or religious figure.

You may imagine this person giving you a message of peace and calm.

[PAUSE]

For the next few minutes or so, let yourself enjoy an imagery story, in whatever way you want. This is very much your story. What special message of peace and calm will you discover? Involve all of your senses. What do you see, feel, and hear?

[PAUSE 2 MINUTES]

[END OF OPTIONAL SEGMENT]

We are about ready to move on.

Gently let go of your story.

[PAUSE 10 SECONDS]

[PAUSE]

How did these exercises make you feel?

TABLE 2.2 *(continued)*

With your eyes closed, ask yourself, how do you feel right now?

If you feel drowsy or sleepy, please raise your right index finger. [RECORD ON BOARD NUMBER OF RESPONSES BY "SLEEPINESS"]

If you feel distant, far away, or detached, raise your finger. [RECORD ON BOARD BY "DISENGAGEMENT"]

If your body feels physically relaxed, loose and limp, maybe your muscles feeling warm and heavy, raise your finger [RECORD BY "PHYSICAL RELAXATION"]

If your mind is quiet, silent, without thought, raise your finger. [RECORD BY "MENTAL QUIET"]

If you feel at ease, at peace, and maybe contented, raise your finger [RECORD BY "MENTAL RELAXATION"]

Do you feel aware, focused, strengthened, or energized? [RECORD BY "STRENGTH AND AWARENESS"]

Do you feel happy or joyful? [RECORD BY "JOY"]

Do you feel loving or thankful? [RECORD BY "LOVE AND PRAYERFUL"]

Do you feel Prayerful, reverent, or spiritual? [RECORD BY "PRAYERFUL"]

And now we continue.

Meditation

Our next exercise is called meditation. It is very simple.

The movement of rocking can be very gentle and peaceful. Gently rocking in a rowboat. Waves gently lap against you. Rocking in a rocking chair on a porch. You are at peace. Nothing is on your mind. You gently rock back and forth, again and again. A hammock. Swinging very gently. Rocking a small child in your arms. There is something very soothing and meditative about simple rocking.

Begin by calmly sitting upright in a comfortable position. Start rocking back and forth in your chair.

[PAUSE]

And now, let each movement become more and more gentle and easy. Let yourself rock effortlessly. Let your body move on its own, in its own way, at its own speed. All you have to do is simply attend.

Let each movement become more and more subtle so that someone watching would barely notice you are rocking. All you have to do

---

(continued)

TABLE 2.2 *(continued)*

is quietly attend to the rocking. Every time your mind wanders, that's okay; gently return to your rocking motion.

For the next minute or so, let your rocking become barely noticeable. And quietly attend.

[PAUSE 60 SECONDS]

Gently let go of what you are attending to. Meditation is a very simple exercise. You simply attend to a simple stimulus. After every distraction, calmly return your attention . . . again and again and again.

If you are like most meditators, your mind wandered. That's OK. Simply return after every distraction.

[PAUSE]

Gently let go of what you are attending to.

With your eyes closed, let a relaxing word, like the word *peace* easily float through your mind. Do not force the word to repeat in any particular way. Simply let the word float by in its own way, at its own volume and speed. All you have to do is gently attend, almost as if you were attending to an echo.

[SPEAK "PEACE" WITH INCREASINGLY QUIET VOICE]

Peace . . . Peace . . . Peace . . . p e a c e.

[PAUSE 60 SECONDS]

[THE FOLLOWING MEDITATION ON A CANDLE FLAME IS RECOMMENDED, BUT OPTIONAL. IF NO CANDLE IS AVAILABLE, SIMPLY GAZE AHEAD, EYES HALF CLOSED]

And now, with your eyes closed, in your mind's eye, imagine a simple spot of light. Perhaps a star, or a candle flame. Or, if you wish, gently open your eyes a little, and attend to the candle in front of you. Calmly attend. Whenever your mind wanders, simply return. There is nothing you have to do or think about.

[PAUSE 60 SECONDS]

[THE FOLLOWING MEDITATION ON A BELL IS RECOMMENDED, BUT OPTIONAL. BEGIN BY RINGING THE BELL ONCE. IF NO BELL IS AVAILABLE, PRESENT SAME INSTRUCTIONS, AND ATTEND TO SOUNDS OF THE PRESENT MOMENT]

And quietly listen to this moment. Let the sounds come and go.

[RING BELL. WAIT 60 SECONDS]

TABLE 2.2 *(continued)*

And now, gently let go of what you are attending to.

[PAUSE]

How did these exercises make you feel?

With your eyes closed, ask yourself, how do you feel right now?

If you feel drowsy or sleepy, please raise your right index finger. [RECORD ON BOARD NUMBER OF RESPONSES BY "SLEEPINESS"]

If you feel distant, far away, or detached, raise your finger. [RECORD ON BOARD BY "DISENGAGEMENT"]

If your body feels physically relaxed, loose and limp, maybe your muscles feeling warm and heavy, raise your finger [RECORD BY "PHYSICAL RELAXATION"]

If your mind is quiet, silent, without thought, raise your finger. [RECORD BY "MENTAL QUIET"]

If you feel at ease, at peace, and maybe contented, raise your finger [RECORD BY "MENTAL RELAXATION"]

Do you feel aware, focused, strengthened, or energized? [RECORD BY "STRENGTH AND AWARENESS"]

Do you feel happy or joyful? [RECORD BY "JOY"]

Do you feel loving or thankful? [RECORD BY "LOVE AND THANKFULNESS"]

Do you feel Prayerful, reverent, or spiritual? [RECORD BY "PRAYERFUL"]

And now we continue.

CONCLUDING DISCUSSION AND PROCESSING

[THE FIRST GROUP QUESTIONS AND PROBES ARE APPROPRIATE FOR INDIVIDUAL CLIENTS AND SMALL GROUPS. USE THE SECOND GROUPS OF PROBES FOR LARGER GROUPS]

Individual Clients and Small Groups

We have just completed three types of relaxation exercise.

(continued)

TABLE 2.2   *(continued)*

In the first part of our tour we tried these exercises:

   Squeezing and Letting Go

   Thinking Warm and Heavy

In the second part we tried these exercises:

   Stretching

   Breathing

And in the third part we enjoyed a special story about a far away place.
And we ended with meditation.

What R-States seem to go with which exercises?

Larger Groups

We have just completed three groups of exercises. How do you feel?

[DISCUSSION]

   What I would like to try now is divide into small teams of three people each. Often after doing Relaxation it can be difficult to explore the exercises and learn from them. People have the tendency to simply sit back and continue relaxing and let everyone else do the discussing. Of course, when everyone does that, there is no discussion!

   First lets break up into teams.

[WAIT FOR TEAMS TO FORM]

   I would like each team to consider these questions:

   Are there differences among relaxation exercises? Which seem to be best for which States?

   What might different exercises be good for? What might different States be good for?

   Let me hand out this Team Worksheet to help.

[DISTRIBUTE HANDOUT FOR EXPERIENTIAL WORKSHOP (pp. 56-57)]

   For the next 15 minutes I would like each team to consider these questions. At then end, we will share our ideas.

[15 MINUTES OF TEAM WORK]

[EACH TEAM DISCUSSES RESPONSES]

TABLE 2.2 *(continued)*

CONCLUSION

I would like to summarize an important point. The key to all forms of relaxation, from professional techniques taught to techniques—yoga and prayer, and simply taking a good vacation—is one simple act: Sustaining passive simple focus. How is this different from what we ordinarily do?

First, everyday life is *effortful*. We plan and strive to achieve our daily goals, anticipate the future, and reflect upon the past. Furthermore, life is moving and changing, it is *discursive* (from the Latin "cursere" for "moving to and fro"). We plan schedules, vacations, and shopping lists; even in idle moments of fantasy, our thoughts ramble from image to image. Discursive effort is good; indeed, it is the very key to success. If you go shopping, you plan which store to go to, how to get there, what to buy, how to pay, and how to get your purchase home. For every single thing you do in life, if you want to succeed or get ahead, you must exert at least some discursive planning effort.

There is one exception. The key to all forms of relaxation is sustained passive simple focus—the opposite of what we usually do to succeed. At first this might seem like a simple thing to do. Everyone has experienced special moments of simple letting go and focusing. Perhaps you were gazing at a sunset, and for an instant golden rays burst through violet clouds. Briefly, you felt deep peace and beauty. Or you may have encountered the secret of simply letting go and simply focusing in relaxing music. Moments of simply focusing and simply letting go are part of life's treasures; but such moments come and go quickly. The sun sets. The music ends. We go on with our day's work. The secret of relaxation is to sustain the moment. This is a very difficult thing to do, something like balancing a basketball on a calm and steady fingertip. Special relaxation techniques, like imagery, yoga, breathing exercises, and meditation, help.

I would like to close this workshop with a question: What is the goal of relaxation? You may learn relaxation for a specific, limited goal, for example, treating a headache or insomnia. This is perfectly fine. But there is more to relaxation than symptom relief. The special act of sustaining passive simple focus can open new doors of understanding. Let me share with you something of a parable, an image taken from modern astronomy. It is an image that also conveys very nicely the promise of relaxation.

One of the most important events in space science has been the launching of the Hubble telescope. Ten times more powerful than

(continued)

TABLE 2.2   *(continued)*

any telescope on earth, the orbiting Hubble can see where no one has seen before. Two things make the Hubble an especially powerful tool. First, it can examine the heavens undistracted by the city lights, haze, and noise of earth. It is above all of that. Second, the Hubble can sustain its focus, unmoved, for hours, days, and even weeks. No earth telescope can do this—shifting continents, passing traffic, changes in the atmosphere, and the rotation of the planet itself mean that the gaze of any land-based telescope is never perfectly steady.

For 10 days in late 1995, astronomers conducted an experiment that changed our vision of the universe. It was a study that had never, and indeed could never have been conducted before. In the "deep field experiment," astronomers aimed the Hubble toward a patch of space that has always appeared completely empty, a small dark spot of sky where earth telescopes indicated nothing existed. (For star gazers, this empty area is close to the handle of the "Big Dipper," and is about one hundredth the size of the moon.) What really exists in this empty space? After a full two weeks of sustained, unmoving focus, the Hubble had a surprising answer—one trillion stars extending to the very edge of the universe. Thousands of galaxies. Each containing billions of stars. Astronomers have concluded that this discovery transforms our vision of the Universe. It is far richer than anyone ever imagined. The deep field experiment shows that what we thought was empty space is filled with an unimaginable richness of stars. And the key to this discovery was sustained passive simple focus. This, as we have seen, is also the key to relaxation.

HANDOUT FOR EXPERIENTIAL WORKSHOP

EXERCISES	R-STATE	GOOD FOR?
Squeeze / Let-Go		
"Warm / Heavy"		
Stretching		
Breathing		
Story Imagery		
Meditation		

TABLE 2.2 *(continued)*

GRAND TOUR EXPERIENTIAL WORKSHOP VARIATIONS

The Grand Tour should be tailored to fit client needs and interests. Here are some ideas for modifying the tour for different populations.

EMPHASIS FOR ACHIEVEMENT-ORIENTED, RESISTANT CLIENTS

Emphasize impact of relaxation exercises on the relaxation response and the potential of relaxation for enhancing strength and productivity (by removing unnecessary distractions and barriers). Focus on PMR, stretching, and breathing. Problematical can be imagery and meditation.

Insight Imagery

You may consider a variety of alternative images, depending on the client group. For example, a group of achievement-oriented, athletic individuals may prefer an image of "skiing down a mountain slope, far away from the cares of the world. At the foot of the hill is an empty cabin, with a message inside."

Meditation

Delete the candle and bell. Describe meditation as an advanced "cognitive focusing training exercise" with demonstrated potential.

EMPHASIS ON STRENGTH, HEALTH, AND HEALING

Emphasize the potential of deep relaxation for enhancing strength, health, and healing. Nearly 2,000 scientific studies, all published in respected peer-reviewed journals, have shown the promise of relaxation-based treatment for over 200 medical disorders. Although relaxation is no cure, it can contribute to other efforts at prevention and recovery. The way relaxation can impact health is still debated. Perhaps by reducing the body's fight or flight "stress response" relaxation reduces the destructive impact of stress. Because stress can impact just about any physical condition, relaxation can have a wide range of benefits. Or perhaps relaxation has a specific impact, with specific techniques im-

(continued)

TABLE 2.2   *(continued)*

pacting specific disorders. One approach may be best for hypertension, another for backaches, and so on.

Variations in Exercise Instructions

Emphasize the potential of each exercise for fostering healing and health. The following phrases can be useful:

Progressive muscle relaxation and autogenic training.

"Let the inner forces of health and healing begin to do their work."

"Let the barriers to health and healing begin to melt away."

"Let the inner work of health and healing take place."

"Let disease and illness begin to dissolve."

Imagery.

"Imagine now, in your minds eye, that you are in a distant place, far from the concerns of the day. This is a place where you are safe and secure. A special place where you can be free from the tensions and concerns that can contribute to illness and disease. This is a special place where the inner forces of strength and health and healing can do their work."

"You can imagine these inner forces in many ways. Perhaps a warm healing energy, like the rays of the sun, or refreshing water from a waterfall, sinks into your skin, slowly melting, dissolving, and washing away disease and illness."

"Perhaps you can imagine healing energy flowing through your veins, bringing life and strength to any part of your body in need. This healing energy flows and slowly carries away poisons and cells that contribute to ill-health."

Stretching.

"Feel the good stretch all along your arm and hand. And reach over your head, pointing to the left. Stretch every inch of your arm and hand. Feel the good energizing sensations as the forces of strength and health and healing are released to do their work."

"Let yourself feel strengthened and energized as inner forces of health and healing are released and do their work."

"Unstretch and bow over, letting tensions and weaknesses flow out of your body into the earth."

"Stretch more and more . . . open yourself up to the energies of life and healing."

"Enjoy the refreshing inner energy as healing forces do their work."

TABLE 2.2 *(continued)*

Breathing.

"As you exhale, let tensions out. Let the forces of weakness and disease and ill health flow out with the air."

"Every breath in brings healing life and energy."

"Every breath out takes with it weakness and tensions and poisons that get in the way of health and healing."

Imagery.

"We are now ready to explore a peaceful and relaxing story, a magical story of strength and health and healing. Imagine you have taken a long and peaceful journey. At the end of your journey you find a special cabin on a pond. You enjoy it with all your senses. You can smell the clean, fresh waters and trees. You hear an occasional dove singing overhead. You feel the refreshing touch of air and sun on your skin. The air is clear and hushed in silent expectation. You begin to look around. The waters of the pond are still like a mirror. The cabin is warm and friendly. In the distance a person is taking a peaceful stroll. This is a wonderful place of healing, one where you can feel fully alive just by being there. This place has a message of peace and wonder for you. It is a special message of strength and health and healing. Perhaps it is just the good feeling of being in such a wonderfully peaceful and pleasant place. Or perhaps a special message, one just for you, appears."

Meditation.

"Our next exercise is called meditation. Meditation is a way of being completely simple and silent inside, so the inner forces of strength and health and healing can work in their own way with complete freedom. In meditation, you become completely quiet, and let inner powers work on their own."

Hypothetical Case Examples

It can be helpful to include some hypothetical cases:

Heart Disease

I would like to begin by sharing a story with you. James is a 63-year-old executive with heart disease. Recently he underwent cardiac surgery. The surgery was successful, but James is very concerned about doing whatever he can to facilitate the healing process, and reduce the processes that contributed to his coronary disease in the first place. His doctor recommended deep relaxation

(continued)

TABLE 2.2   *(continued)*

as part of a larger treatment and prevention plan that includes changes in diet, exercise, and work stress. James has already chosen to stop smoking. Research suggests that deep relaxation can facilitate the physical healing process. Also, we know that stress directly contributes to hardening of the arteries, a serious contributor to heart disease, and that relaxation can for many significantly reduce stress.

However, James also knows that different approaches to relaxation have quite different effects. His job is to find what truly works for him.

Cancer

Beatrice has just had surgery for breast cancer. The surgery was successful, but she wants to do whatever she can to help recover and reduce the processes that may have contributed to cancer in the first place. Her doctor recommended deep relaxation as part of a larger treatment and prevention plan that includes changes in diet, exercise, and work stress. Beatrice has already chosen to stop smoking. Research suggests that deep relaxation can facilitate the physical healing process. Also, we know that stress can directly contribute lowered resistance, or impaired immune system functioning, and it is the body's resistance that helps prevent and fight off cancer. Relaxation can for many significantly reduce stress. However, Beatrice also knows that different approaches to relaxation have quite different effects. Her job is to find what truly works for her.

Allergies

Chris suffers from a variety of allergies. Her problem is most severe in the summer and fall. Her physician prescribed a number of medications, but all have side effects. An allergy specialist noted that often allergies are aggravated by stress and changes in the immune system. Deep relaxation can for some reduce stress and moderate the impact of allergies. Chris wants to explore a variety of techniques to find which work best for her.

SUBSTANCE ABUSE CLIENTS

Emphasize the potential of deep relaxation in substance abuse and recovery programs.

"How can deep relaxation training help people free themselves from the compulsions of tobacco, alcohol, and drug abuse? First,

TABLE 2.2 *(continued)*

by giving a tool for blocking initial cravings. A big problem for those trying to stop smoking, drinking, or using drugs is relapse. That is, getting hooked again. You can help prevent relapse by learning to identify early cravings, and then practicing a quick and simple deep relaxation technique to cool down the cravings."

"There is a second, perhaps more powerful way deep relaxation training can help. The Relaxation states you learn can provide a very satisfying substitute for the seductive rewards of tobacco, alcohol, and drugs. People often use substances to evoke pleasurable states of mind. Exciting recent research shows that we have the capacity of producing similar relaxation states of mind on our own, without the use of chemicals. The brain is a remarkable organ. Special chemicals, some called endorphins and neurotransmitters can actually trigger very rewarding states of mind. And the techniques of deep relaxation training can give you healthy and natural tools for doing this."

SPIRITUAL MEDITATION AND SELF-EXPLORATION

Provide a spiritual or meditative orientation:
"In this workshop we will be taking a look at a powerful spiritual tool. Meditation. As you may know, meditation can be used in may ways, in psychotherapy and stress management for treating anxiety and phobias. It's used in medicine for pain management, preparation for surgery, recovery from surgery, managing the side effects of chemotherapy. Artists use it to enhance creativity, athletes to improve their game, and business executives to increase productivity. Although all of these uses are important, we will explore the spiritual use of meditation for self-exploration."

TRADITIONAL WESTERN RELIGION (JUDAISM, CHRISTIANITY, ISLAM, ETC.)

Emphasize how standard professional deep relaxation exercises are in themselves completely neutral, like other tools such as books and music:
"At this point it is important to consider a problem some people have. Is it right to incorporate relaxation exercises into something as serious as prayer? First, it is important to realize that each of these exercises have been used in religions around the world as part of prayer. They do not belong to any one religion, but are used by all. You might think of the tools of relaxation

(continued)

TABLE 2.2 *(continued)*

like other tools we use in religion, reading books, singing songs, making beautiful art. Each of these tools is used in all world religions as part of prayer and worship. No one religion owns the idea of using books, song, or arts. These are neutral tools. So to are the tools of deep relaxation training. They belong to no one religion, but can be applied in all."

You can include specific exercise variations:

Progressive Muscle Relaxation.

"Let's begin by attending to our shoulder muscles. While keeping the rest of your body loose and relaxed, shrug your shoulders *now!* Create a nice, good squeeze. Feel it throughout your shoulder muscles. This is how we hold on to our worries and concerns."

"Now let go! Let yourself go completely limp."

"As you relax, give your tension to God."

"Begin to sink into a pleasant state of relaxation, safe in the hands of God."

"Let's try that once again. Focus your attention on your shoulder muscles. And shrug them *now!* Create a nice, good shrug. This is how we tightly cling to our cares and concerns."

"And let go. Go completely limp."

"Let the tension begin to flow away to God."

"Trust God as your muscles begin to feel more limp and loose."

"Let yourself sink deeper and deeper into relaxation, into the safe and loving hands of God."

Autogenic Training.

"Let yourself continue to sink deeper and deeper into relaxation.
Far away from the cares and concerns of the day.
There is nothing you have to do.
You are in God's gentle, caring hands, safe and secure.
And quietly attend to your hands.
Let the words, "warm and heavy" float through your mind, like echoes.
Let these words simply float over and over, at a very slow and lazy pace. There is nothing you have to do. Let your body relax and feel warm and heavy. You are safely in the hands of God."

Sense Imagery.

Present images that are simple passive religious environments, a peaceful pasture outside a country chapel, a temple garden, a warm pond outside a mosque.

TABLE 2.2 *(continued)*

Stretching.

"Lift your arms and hands over your head and reach to the heavens, all the way."

"Make your stretch full and complete, as if you are celebrating the glories of God's world."

"Let both arms hang to your sides."

"And slowly begin to bow forward, as if you were bowing in prayer and worship."

Breathing Exercises.

"Attend to the breath of life."

"The air God gives us every moment of every day."

"The life and energy God gives us every moment of every day."

Insight Imagery.

Suggest a story with religious implications, a journey to a religious retreat or house of a religious leader.

Meditation.

Rename this exercise "silent prayer."

"We end with an exercise called silent prayer. These are prayers in which we do not speak. In fact we do nothing but become completely still. Completely silent. So the spirit of God can flow. Silent prayers are very very simple."

"Select a mantra or visual image that fits in one's religious tradition."

TABLE 2.3   Behavioral Signs of Relaxation Rating Scale

Below are a number of behavioral signs of relaxation. Indicate how well each fits or describes the person you are rating. Do this by putting a number in the space to the left of each statement. Please use the following scale:

How well does the item you are reading fit the person you are rating?

1 = Fits Not at All
2 = Fits Slightly
3 = Fits Moderately
4 = Fits Very Well
5 = Fits Extremely Well

Breathing

_____   1. Slow breathing pace
_____   2. Even breathing rhythm
_____   3. Greater use of diaphragm (stomach rising and falling)
_____   4. Reduced chest extension

Posture

_____   5. Shoulders sloped
_____   6. Head slightly tilted
_____   7. Limbs and other body parts are in open, relaxed position
              a. jaws slightly parted
              b. palms open
              c. fingers curled and not straight or clenched
              d. knees and feet pointing apart

Muscle Activity

_____   8. Little restless movement
              a. eyes closed; no blinking, looking around, staring
              b. palms open
              c. no chewing, biting lips, swallowing
_____   9. Little clenching and bracing
_____   10. Face, neck, arms, and hands are smooth and unwrinkled with
              no sign of twitching or extended veins or muscles.

Scoring key: Simply add the ratings for each section

TABLE 2.4 Unidimensional Self-Report Measures of Stress Arousal and Symptoms

Measure	Symptoms/State
Beck Depression Inventory (Beck, Ward, Mendelson, Mock, & Erbaugh, 1961)	Depression (anxiety and hostility versions also available)
State-Trait Anxiety Inventory (Spielberger, Gorsuch, & Lushene, 1970)	Anxiety (hostility version also available)
Center for Epidemiologic Studies Depression Scales (Radloff, 1977)	Depressed affect, positive affect, interpersonal problems, somatic problems
Profile of Mood States (McNair, Lorr, & Dropplemann, 1971)	Tension-anxiety, depression-dejection, confusion, anger-hostility, vigor, fatigue

TABLE 2.5 Words Associated with Various R-States

These words have at one time or another correlated with the listed R-States. If a relaxation client reports experiencing any of the listed words, one might hypothesize that he or she is experiencing the associated R-State and may readily experience the other words in that group. A relaxation trainer may consider introducing the other words into a relaxation script as suggestions in order to enhance the associated R-State.

Sleepiness (Sleepy)
    Key words: *Dozing off, napping, drowsy, sleepy*

Disengagement (disengaged)
    Key words: *Distant, far away, indifferent, detached*
    Additional words:
        Dissolving (also Physical Relaxation)
        Escaped
        Forgetting what one is doing, where one is (what was being said, going on around)
        Heavy (also Physical Relaxation)
        Loss of sensation in parts of body (hands, feet, etc.)
        Passive
        Sinking (also Physical Relaxation)

Mental Quiet (Mentally Quiet)
    Key content: *Mind is quiet, without thought; inner stillness, not thinking about anything*
    Additional words:
        Speechless (also Disengagement)
        Without words
        Silent

(continued)

TABLE 2.5   *(continued)*

Physical Relaxation (Physically Relaxed)
  Key words: *Warm, heavy, limp*
  Additional words:
    Dissolving (also Disengagement)
    Deep (as in "going deeper; also Disengagement)
    Elastic
    Floating (also Disengagement)
    Light
    Liquid
    Listless (also Sleepiness)
    Massaged
    Melting
    Motionless
    Sinking
    Slack
    Slow
    Supple
    Throbbing
    Tingling

Mental Relaxation (Mentally Relaxed)
  Key words: *At ease, at peace, contented*
  Additional words:
    Calm
    Carefree
    Laid back
    Relaxed
    Relieved
    Rested
    Restored
    Refreshed
    Soothed

Strength and Awareness (Strengthened and Aware)
  Key words: *Aware, focused clear, energized, confident, strengthened*
  Additional words
    Alive
    Awake
    Creative (also Joy)

Joy (Joyful)
  Key words: *Joy, happiness*
  Additional words:
    Beautiful (also Prayerful)
    Blessed (also Prayerful)
    Childlike

TABLE 2.5 *(continued)*

Complete
Creative (also Strength and Awareness)
Delighted
Fascinated
Free
Fun
Glorious
Glowing
Harmonious
Healing
Hopeful
Infinite (also Prayerful)
Inspired (also Prayerful)
Knowing (also Prayerful)
Loving (also Love and Thankfulness)
Optimistic (also Strength and Awareness)
Playful
Pleased
Sensuous
Spontaneous
Thankful (also Love and Thankfulness)
Timeless (also Prayerful)
Trusting
Understanding (also Prayerful)
Warm (also Physical Relaxation)
Whole
Wonderful

Love and Thankfulness (loving and thankful)
  Key words: *Love, thankful*
  Additional words:
    Caring
    Compassionate
    Grateful

Prayerfulness (Prayerful)
  Key words: *Prayerful, reverent, spiritual*
  Additional words:
    Answered
    Awe-filled
    Blessed (also Joy)
    Cleansed
    Cosmic
    Eternal
    Knowing (also Joy)

(continued)

TABLE 2.5   *(continued)*

Mysterious (also Disengagement)
Mystical (also Disengagement)
Reborn
Understanding (also Joy)
Selfless
Surrendering
Wonder, sense of
Worshipful

TABLE 2.6   Finger Signal System for Assessing R-States

[INTRODUCTION] When we relax, from time to time I may ask how you are feeling. In order not to disturb your relaxation, we will use a simple signal system. If I were to ask "Do you feel relaxed?" simply raise your right index finger, like this [DEMONSTRATE] if this is indeed how you feel. If this is not how you feel, just remain still. Let's try this. Do you understand these instructions? If you do, please raise your right index finger now. [CHECK TO SEE IF CLIENT IS RESPONDING.]

With your eyes closed, ask yourself, how do you feel right now?

[SLEEPINESS]

If you feel drowsy or sleepy, please raise your right index finger.

[DISENGAGEMENT]

If you feel distant, far away, or detached, raise your finger.

[PHYSICAL RELAXATION]

If your body feels physically relaxed, loose and limp, maybe your muscles feeling warm and heavy, raise your finger.

[MENTAL QUIET]

If your mind is quiet, silent, without thought, raise your finger.

[MENTAL RELAXATION]

If you feel at ease, at peace, and maybe contented, raise your finger.

[STRENGTH AND AWARENESS]

Do you feel aware, focused, strengthened, or energized?

[JOY]

Do you feel happy or joyful?

[LOVE AND THANKFULNESS]

Do you feel loving or thankful?

[PRAYERFULNESS]

Do you feel prayerful, reverent, or spiritual?

TABLE 2.7   Script for Reviewing Possible Goals of Relaxation

What are your goals of relaxation training? Perhaps one of the simplest uses is for tension "spot relief." If you can identify a problem or discomfort in a specific part of the body, often a specific relaxation technique can be found that might be useful when applied to this part.

Researchers have found that people learn relaxation for the following reasons (show client list):

Medical

Preparing for or recovering from surgery

Managing anxiety over medical/dental procedures

Managing the side effects of prescription medication.

Managing physical symptoms.

Substance Abuse/Compulsive Behavior

Controlling tobacco use

Controlling use of illegal substances

Controlling eating problems

Dealing with compulsive behavior

Psychological Distress

Managing anxiety, worry, and frustration

Managing depression

Increasing productivity

Reducing stress

Creativity

Enhancing artistic work

Enhancing creativity

Enhancing personal insight

General Health

Enhancing resistance to disease.

Enhancing physical health

Increasing personal strength or stamina

Enhancing personal alertness and energy.

Enhancing ability to meditate

Pain/Sleep

Dealing with insomnia

(continued)

TABLE 2.7   *(continued)*

Enhancing sleep

Reducing pain and discomfort.

Athletics/Sex

Preparing for or recovering from exercise workouts

Enhancing sex

Enhancing my performance at sports

Spiritual Growth

Developing ability to pray

Spiritual growth

Interpersonal Stress

Enhancing ability to cope with others

Dealing with interpersonal conflict

Maybe you already do a relaxation technique and want to make it work better. Is that your goal?

Whatever your goals, it is important to keep a number of precautions in mind.

1.   Relaxation is not a cure-all. Many of its possible uses have yet to be demonstrated. Relaxation is not a substitute for other legitimate treatments, although it can supplement many. This is important to recognize because many popularized relaxation programs tend to oversell what they offer. However, it can be helpful to try relaxation in a spirit of open-minded experimentation. Try it and see what happens.

2.   Relaxation effects are not immediate. It takes time to develop relaxation skills.

3.   There are many approaches to relaxation. What works for you may not work for others. If an approach does not work for you, try another.

What are your goals?

3

Basic Instructions for the Six Major Approaches to Relaxation

In this chapter we present formal instructions for six major approaches to relaxation: progressive muscle relaxation (PMR), autogenic training (AT), breathing exercises, stretching exercises, imagery, and meditation. We restrict ourselves to those exercises that have been widely applied, both in research and in professional practice. Exercises are presented in an order I have found most useful for client mastery. Before proceeding to formal relaxation, we consider a simple and inexpensive preparatory exercise that for many clients may provide sufficient relaxation—taking time off.

The instructions in this chapter are flexible and can be used in various ways. I teach clients all techniques in the order presented, and then make an individualized relaxation tape using the instructions in chapter 4. This takes 10–12 weeks. It is possible to present single approaches and even combine one or two, for example, breathing and meditation or AT and imagery. Brief Relaxation Training (chapter 5) presents all 6 approaches in a single session.

However a technique is presented, I recommend the following five steps:

Step 1: Explanation and rationale. Explain what a technique is and how it works. The explanation and rationale should be viewed as an essential part of relaxation training, even contributing to relaxation itself. In it here that a client is motivated to practice and can bring up questions and concerns.

Step 2: Demonstration. Model the specifics of each exercise to be presented, invite the client to try, and then fine-tune the exercise if problems arise. For example, a full yoga sequence might include a hand stretch, arm stretch, back stretch, neck stretch, and so on. In the demonstration phase, the client learns one component of an exercise sequence, perhaps the hand stretch. The trainer models, the client tries the exercise out, and the trainer makes corrections. If it is clear the client has mastered the hand stretch, training proceeds to the next exercise in the sequence, the arm stretch in this case. In the demonstration phase, an entire exercise sequence is disassembled and taught in parts. Once each part is mastered, proceed to dress rehearsal.

Step 3: Dress rehearsal.   Both the trainer and client proceed through an entire relaxation sequence, without interruption, just as the client will do away from training.

Step 4: Checking.   After dress rehearsal, check the level of relaxation using the Behavioral Signs of Relaxation Rating Scale (Table 2.3) and the Smith Relaxation States Inventory (Appendix). Ask if any problems emerged.

Step 5: Modification.   Modify the sequence if necessary to enhance relaxation and reduce problems.

Finally, for each approach, I offer conservative suggestions as to how techniques might be used. I cannot urge too strongly that these tabular applications should be used as tentative suggestions, not prescriptions.

SETTING TIME ASIDE FOR REST

Before considering the six major approaches to professional relaxation, we consider a relaxation strategy that is especially easy and economical. For some clients, it is sufficient for reaching relaxation goals. It also helps demonstrate the idea of R-States and R-Beliefs. The technique simply involves scheduling a time every day for completing any activity the client finds quietly relaxing. Details for this approach are adapted from Smith (1987).

Step 1: Rationale

Explain to clients that the most difficult problem that beginners have with relaxation training is learning to set aside a specific daily time for relaxation. This might seem like an easy thing to do, but it is important not to underestimate the difficulties. There are many hidden forces that can get in the way. First, our society has a deep and often hidden prejudice against inactivity and rest. Relaxation is associated with laziness and wasting time. Society tells us it is OK to take it easy *after* we have completed our work. In fact, rest can be just as important and meaningful as work. Second, we often have the mistaken belief that success must always be preceded by strain and toil. It can take time to see that rest-related skills are also important.

There is a third, more insidious resistance as well. People with a high-stress pattern of living may actually become accustomed to and perhaps even crave a chronic, high level of stress arousal. Just as the alcoholic craves alcohol when sober, the "stressoholic" craves stressful activity even when at rest.

When clients begin practicing a relaxation technique, they may well experience the combined effects of society's pressures and their own stress addiction. They may feel impatient, bored, and restless. They may want things to happen immediately.

Setting time aside for rest is a formal relaxation technique designed to counter some of the many sources of resistance to relaxation. Through the behavioral procedure of shaping, a client is taught to tolerate regular time-off periods of quiet by incorporating a pleasurable and simple relaxing activity that he or she already knows. Such an activity also has the effect of reinforcing the healthy habit of taking time off.

Steps 2, 3, 4, and 5: Demonstration, Dress Rehearsal, Checking, Modification

Because of the simplicity of the time-off approach, we can combine the demonstration, dress rehearsal, checking, and modification stages. The next phase of training involves selecting a proper relaxation activity and time. Elsewhere, I offer guidelines (Smith, 1987). See Table 3.1 at end of chapter.

Often, clients will have great difficulty thinking of pleasant, quiet things to do. Perhaps this itself is a sign of stress addiction. I "prime the pump" by inviting them to brainstorm with me. Try to think of as many activities as possible. Possible activities include

Crafts (simple)

Daydreaming

Doing one's nails

Doodling

Knitting

Listening to quiet music

Looking at collected postcards or stamps

Looking out the window

Reading a magazine

Reading a novel

Playing a simple musical instrument just for fun

Sewing

Next, select a proper time-off time. Ask clients to suggest a workable time each day, as you record. Then discuss the selected times. Play "devil's advocate" and see if you can uncover some hidden problems. For example, do not select a time that is within 1 hour after eating. During that interval, blood is directed to the stomach for digestion, and your client may not fully benefit from relaxation. Do not select a time in which the possibility of interruption is high. For example, if a client talks with friends in early evening, it would not be a good idea to select this time for practicing relaxation. Finally, a client should not select a time when there is urgent unfinished business to complete. It is difficult to relax when thinking about other things to do. Remind your clients that time off is a special time, just for them.

Finally, select a time-off place, one that is quiet and free from interruption. The place should be relatively free from outside stimulation, that is, dimly lit, few noises, a comfortable chair, and so on. A client may wish to enhance a relaxation place by introducing art or objects suggestive of relaxation.

APPROACH 1: PROGRESSIVE MUSCLE RELAXATION

PMR is perhaps the most popular formal professional approach to relaxation in the West. The basic strategy is to systematically tense up and then release tension in various muscle groups (alternate forms involve just releasing tension without first creating tension). PMR is relatively familiar and unthreatening, particularly well suited for evoking R-States of Sleepiness, Disengagement, Physical Relaxation, and Mental Relaxation, but it may be ill-suited for the R-States Mental Quiet, Strength and Awareness, Joy, Love and Thankfulness, and Prayerfulness (Smith, 1999). PMR also is valuable for clients who have difficulty relaxing or maintaining focus on a relaxation task because of anxiety (Weinstein & Smith, 1992), impulsivity, or cognitive impairment. I disagree with Bernstein and Carlson (1993), who suggest not using PMR for clients who have difficulty focusing attention; indeed, PMR may be one of the most appropriate approaches to relaxation for such clients. The most direct clinical applications are for disorders with a clear muscle-tension component. The somatic specificity model (see *ABC Relaxation Theory*) recommends targeting skeletal muscle groups that may be sources of tension. See Table 3.2 (at end of chapter) for clinical applications suggested by others.

Care should be taken in applying PMR tension-release exercises to parts of the body where organs, muscles, bones, or connective tissues are injured, weak, compromised by illness, or recovering from surgery. The same applies for clients who display a loss of voluntary muscular control due to neuromuscular disability. Often PMR is not appropriate for parts of the body that suffer from chronic pain or discomfort. Indeed, for certain parts of the body, particularly the lower back, muscle strengthening may be more appropriate than targeted relaxation. In general, if there is any question about applying PMR to a specific muscle group, that group should be omitted from a training sequence.

We shall consider three variations of PMR, overt, minimal, and covert. They can be presented independently, or in sequence (with 2–3 weeks devoted to each) depending on client preferences. By far, the most widely applied version is overt PMR.

Overt PMR

Step 1: Explanation and Rationale

Explain the importance of muscle tension in stress and anxiety. One goal of PMR is to induce muscle relaxation by creating its opposite; one first tenses up, and then releases tension. Because clients may find this paradoxical, explain how initially tensing up may actually help the process of tension release through something of a "rebound effect." The image of a pendulum can help. To make a pendulum swing in one direction, one could push it in that direction. Another way would be to pull it in the opposite direction, building up tension and then letting go. The built-up energy is released as the pendulum swings in the opposite direction. Other metaphors can be used to illustrate the hypothetical rebound effect, including pushing a sled up a snowy hill and letting go so that it can slide down and pulling an arrow back on the string of a bow and then releasing tension, letting the arrow soar.

Illustrate the overt tension-release act on the shoulder muscles: "Here is how we will tense up and let go. Let me demonstrate on the shoulders. First, let's shrug our shoulders and create a good squeeze. Do this now, with me. Let the tension build. Now let go. Let the tension flow. Simply let the tightness dissolve and begin to melt away. There is nothing you have to do but relax. There, how was that? We will be tensing up and releasing all the major muscle groups in the body."

Step 2: Demonstration

In this phase, demonstrate tensing up and letting go for every muscle group. Two popular sequences have been presented by Smith (1987) and Bernstein and Carlson (1993). I present both in Table 3.3 (end of chapter) to illustrate an important principle—there are several ways of achieving a tense-release effect. This table gives you several strategies to try. In the demonstration phase, explore with your client different approaches until you find what works.

When presenting overt PMR, I find these procedural rules helpful:

1. *Posture.* It is preferable to practice with eyes closed (except when looking at a trainer modeling). Avoid an upright alert position that fosters R-States related to opening up. Also, avoid crossing or extending the arms or legs, positions that can generate distracting tension. PMR can be practiced while seated in a soft, comfortable lounge chair. One might assume a position often recommended by autogenic trainers: the client sits comfortably with arms resting easily in the lap and head slightly bowed (not so much as to cut off breathing). This position resembles that of a seated string puppet, with strings cut so that the puppet is seated relaxed, limp, and slightly slouched. PMR can be practiced in a reclining position, although such a position can foster the R-State Sleepiness.

2. *Double practice.* For each muscle group, present a complete tense–let go cycle twice ("Make a fist . . . let go . . . make a fist . . . let go").

3. *Separate practice for left and right side.* For arms, hands, legs, and feet, practice a complete cycle ("tense–let go . . . tense–let go") twice on the right side and then twice on the left side of the body.

4. *Frequent relaxation checks.* After presenting a tense–let go cycle twice and before moving on to the next muscle group, ask the client if he or she is relaxed (by gently shaking head "yes" or "no"). If not relaxed, repeat the exercise up to three more times. A special arm exercise relaxation check can be a useful demonstration of the idea of muscle relaxation. After a client has tensed and relaxed the right arm, simply lift the relaxed arm about 5 inches and let it drop. If the arm stays in the air or descends slowly, then it is not relaxed. A relaxed arm should drop with an audible thud, like a dropped piece of meat. Use these instructions for this arm exercise relaxation check:

"In a minute I'm going to do a simple little check. I will gently hold your wrist like this (demonstrate on your own wrist) and lift your arm a few inches and let it drop. That's all. Ready? Make sure your arm is completely relaxed. Now I gently hold your wrist. [HOLD CLIENT'S WRIST.] I lift it up. [LIFT ARM.] And I let go. [LET IT DROP. IF ARM DROPS SLOWLY OR STAYS UP, EXPLAIN HOW THIS ILLUS-TRATES THAT THERE IS STILL MUSCLE TENSION. DEMON-STRATE HOW THE ARM SHOULD DROP, AND TRY AGAIN ONE OR TWO TIMES.]

5. *The "keep talking" rule.* PMR appears to work best for clients who are very tense and have a hard time focusing. The trainer makes focusing easier through continuous and monotonous relaxation talk, or patter.

6. *The 2–4 rule.* Trainer patter instructs a client either to tense up or let go. Generally, speak two "tense up" phrases followed by four "let go" phrases. This will result in a properly timed sequence (i.e., 5 or so seconds for the tense-up phase and 20–30 seconds for the let-go phase). In the let-go phase, a 3–5 second pause should precede each statement.

7. *The PMR voice.* Pay very close attention to voice speed, volume, and quality. Beginning instructors talk too fast and do not introduce enough pauses. Cultivate a different voice for speaking tense-up and let-go phases. Tense-up talk should be relatively loud and tense, as if you were a gym coach urging your students to put forth more effort. Let-go talk should communicate letting go. The first let-go phrase (of the four) should be spoken with a sigh, almost as if you were letting go—"And let go-o-o-o." The remaining phrases should be spoken slowly and softly,

in a rather gentle and uninteresting monotone. It is difficult for most beginning instructors to deploy an appropriately monotonous PMR let-go voice. It should sound something like a tape recording that has been deliberately slowed or like the voice of someone who is dozing off. Strive for a slow, soft, and boring tone of voice.

8. *What to say.* No PMR script ever won a literary award. Because of the requirement to keep talking, PMR is necessarily uninteresting and repetitive. I suggest selecting tense-up and let-go phrases from the menu shown in Table 3.4 at the end of the chapter. Note that there are seven topics that let-go phrases can reflect: (a) the process of releasing tension; (b) reassurances of control; (c) suggestions of R-States of Disengagement, Physical Relaxation, and to some extent, Mental Relaxation; (d) suggestions of cognitive tension relief; (e) suggestions of somatic tension relief; (f) phrases discriminating tension and tension relief; and (g) phrases of increased generalization of relaxation.

Although beginners often find it difficult to remember what to say in PMR, I recommend not reading a PMR script. It is important to observe client nonverbal cues for signs of when an exercise is or is not working. Instead, I recommend two tools for novice instructors: (1) memorize the 11 muscle groups targeted in PMR (Table 3.5); (2) place a list of let-go phrases on one's lap or nearby table (Table 3.6) to suggest patter. Remember: it is important to continue talking; boring repetition is okay.

9. *Avoid words suggesting R-States of Strength and Awareness, Joy, Love and Thankfulness, and Prayerfulness.* Again, PMR is an eminent technique of Disengagement and Physical Relaxation. In addition, avoid words suggesting Mental Relaxation that can also indirectly suggest awareness ("peaceful, rest, refreshment, contentment, restored"). Such words can be introduced at the end of training to enhance a desired aftereffect.

10. *Suggest increased generalization of relaxation as session progresses.* Early in the session, restrict your instructions to specific body parts. However, when the session is at least half over, begin to introduce phrases suggesting generalization to the entire body.

11. *Terminate the session.* Use a special phrase for ending the session. I use "And let go of what you are attending to. We have completed our relaxation session. Slowly open your eyes and take a deep breath."

Step 3: Dress Rehearsal

Present instructions for the entire PMR script, from beginning to end, without stop. You can present them live (don't read them) or play a tape of the script in Table 3.5. If you present instructions live, you can tape them at the same time. If you play a tape, practice along with your client.

Step 4: Checking

Check for any problems that have emerged. Some of the more common problems include the following.

Clients may complain of cramps. If a muscle cramps, do not include it in the sequence. The trainer should not show alarm or upset when a cramp occurs. Wait patiently, and the cramp will most likely go away. It is OK for a client to massage or rub a cramped muscle or simply shift to a comfortable position in which little strain is placed on the muscle (the trainer should not touch the client).

A client may giggle or appear to cry in a relaxation session. Such reactions are often a sign of tension release. The trainer should simply ignore them, not displaying any concern or upset. If necessary, reassure the client: "Tears may come to your eyes. That's OK. We can continue."

A client may complain of an inability to create muscle tension. Try alternative methods of tensing up until an effect is created. If this doesn't work, isolate separate muscles and target them. For example, if a client has difficulty creating tension in the face, try focusing on the forehead, then the cheeks and nose, and then the lower face, as suggested in Table 3.3 (end of chapter). Exercises targeting the lower back and abdomen are less likely to create vivid feelings of tension.

A client may complain of an inability to release tension. In these cases repeat the tense–let go cycle, for a total of no more than five times.

Clients may report drowsiness or may fall asleep in training. Drowsiness is normal; it can be an indication of the R-States Sleepiness or Disengagement. However, frequent sleep during practice should be avoided. If you suspect that a client has fallen asleep and he is not displaying the usual obvious signs (snoring), check for consciousness. Bernstein and Borkovec (1973) suggest repeating the relaxation check, "Let me know if you are relaxed." If the client does not respond, repeat a tense–let go cycle. If a client does not respond, wait 10 seconds and repeat it again, louder. Continue until the client awakens.

If sleepiness is a persistent problem, make sure that no external factors are contributing (eating, drinking, or taking drugs or medication before practice; practicing in a poorly ventilated room; practicing in bed; practicing at a time generally reserved for sleep). If the problem persists, PMR can be modified to increase the level of stimulation (practicing in a cooler room; turning up the lights; presenting instructions in a louder voice; having the client sit upright in a less comfortable chair; including client-selected background music; practicing with eyes open; including engaging instructions to focus on relaxation patter and muscle sensations; including words suggesting R-States Mental Relaxation or Strength and Awareness. You may include a few stretches or breathing exercises to cultivate wake-fulness. See general discussion of sleepiness at the end of this chapter.

Step 5: Modification

Change or delete exercises when necessary.

Minimal and Covert PMR

Jacobson's original PMR technique involved tensing up very slightly before letting go. The emphasis was on detecting increasingly subtle levels of tension before releasing it. In spite of the nearly universal acceptance of overt PMR among PMR practitioners, the relative superiority of one approach over another has yet to be demonstrated. Highly anxious clients or those who are easily distracted may need overt tension-release cycles to maintain attention on the relaxation task.

Typically, as a client gains skill at relaxing (usually in 2 or 3 weeks of daily practice), muscle groups can be combined—for example, hands, arms, and shoulders; face and neck; shoulders, chest, and stomach; and legs, calves, and feet. In addition, for limbs, both right and left sides can be practiced simultaneously. When a client can achieve relaxation with combined muscle groups (3 or 4 weeks), covert procedures can be attempted.

Three covert systems are available. A popular version involves in-structing clients to attend systematically to each muscle group targeted, notice any feelings of tension, and simply let go of tension without first tightening up (Bernstein & Carlson, 1993). An alternative has the client look for tension with every incoming breath and release tension with every exhalation (Smith, 1987). Trainers can adapt the instruction script in Table 3.5 by simply deleting the "tense up–let go now" instructions. For clients who dislike actively tensing up, this version of covert PMR can be an appropriate starting point.

Third, the above covert sequence can be terminated with a relaxation cue, for example, deep breathing, an image, or a verbal countdown. Eventually, this cue can be used in itself to evoke relaxation. I consider this third approach to be an example of bridging different families of relaxation and will consider it more fully later on. Unfortunately, PMR instruction books give little or no consideration of what words are appro-priate relaxation cues. I suggest any words suggesting the R-States Disengagement or Physical Relaxation and possibly Mental Relaxation and Sleepiness (especially if PMR is to be used to treat insomnia). Words suggesting increased awareness or affect ("peaceful," "refreshed") are not appropriate, given that they suggest R-States contrary to what PMR tends to evoke. Of course, selection of a relaxation cue should be a collaborative effort between client and trainer.

The following are suggestions for enhancing PMR:

- Breathe in before tensing up; exhale while releasing tension.
- Follow each tense–let go cycle with a stretch of the same muscle group ("Tense and let go of your right hand; stretch and unstretch your right hand").
- Incorporate autogenic "warm and heavy" suggestions.
- Incorporate imagery suggestive of Physical Relaxation, or the release of tension ("Let tension unwind like a tight wad of paper," "melt away like candle wax").
- Suggest casual everyday relaxation activities that might also contribute to the R-States Physical Relaxation, Disengagement, and possibly Sleepiness. Examples include hot baths, sun bathing, and massage.

TABLE 3.5   Sample Script for Overt PMR

(Words that are in **boldface** or [BRACKETED] are special instructions to trainers. These words are not to be read or spoken to clients. Between each phrase, wait 2 full seconds. Mentally count "one thousand one . . . one thousand two.")

Right Hand

Let's begin by focusing on the right hand.

Squeeze the fingers together by making a fist, now.

Tighten up the muscles.

Let the tension grow.

And let go.

Release the tension.

Let your muscles begin to go limp.

Let the tension begin to flow out.

(continued)

TABLE 3.5 *(continued)*

As your hand sinks into relaxation.

Right Hand (Repeat)

Once again, make a fist with the right hand now.

Keep the rest of your body relaxed.

Let the tension grow.

Let it build.

And let go.

Let the muscles go limp.

There is nothing you have to do.

Let the tension begin to flow away.

Sink into relaxation.

Left Hand

This time focus on the left hand.

Make a tight fist with your left hand, now.

Let the tension grow.

And let go.

Let the tension flow out.

Feelings of tension dissolve.

Become more limp and loose.

Let yourself relax.

Left Hand (Repeat)

Once again, squeeze up the left hand, now.

Squeeze the muscles more and more.

Keep the rest of your body relaxed.

Let the tension feel satisfying and complete.

And let go.

Let your tension begin to unwind.

TABLE 3.5 *(continued)*

As you relax, your muscles become more and more loose.

Let yourself forget the tensions and cares of the world.

Right Arm

This time focus on your right arm.

Squeeze your lower and upper arm together, touching your shoulder with your wrist. Do this now.

Press tighter and tighter.

Notice the feelings of tension.

And let go.

Let the tension go.

Let the rest of your body remain relaxed.

The tension melts away.

Let the muscles become more deeply relaxed.

Right Arm (Repeat)

Again, squeeze your lower and upper arm together, now.

Don't tense up so it hurts.

Tense up only the muscles of the arm.

And let go.

Let your muscles go limp.

As you relax, your muscles become more loose.

You sink deeper into relaxation.

Far away from the cares of the world.

Left Arm

And, the left arm. Tighten it up now.

Tighten up the muscles.

Let the tension build.

And let go.

(continued)

TABLE 3.5 *(continued)*

Let the muscles begin to smooth out.

Let your tension begin to unwind.

Let the tension flow out.

Let yourself sink deeper and deeper into relaxation.

Left Arm (Repeat)

Again, tense up the left arm, now.

Let the feelings of tightness grow

Let the muscles get nice and hard.

And let go.

Let tension dissolve.

The tension begins to flow away.

There is nothing you have to do.

Right Arm and Side

This time, rest your hand in your lap.

Focus your attention on your arm and side and press them together, now.

Tighten up the muscles.

Let the tension grow.

And let go.

Let the muscles go completely limp.

Let tension flow away.

Let yourself relax.

Right Arm and Side (Repeat)

Again tighten up your right arm and side, now.

Let your muscles become more tight.

Let the tension grow.

And let go.·

Let your muscles go completely limp.

Let tension flow.

TABLE 3.5 *(continued)*

Sink more and more deeply into relaxation.

Left Arm and Side

Tighten up your left arm and side, now.

Let the feelings of tightness grow.

Let the tension feel satisfying and complete.

And let go.

Release the tension.

Let the muscles become more and more limp.

As you relax, your muscles become more and more heavy.

Left Arm and Side (Repeat)

Again, tighten up your left arm and side, now.

Let the tension grow.

Feel the tension.

And let go.

Begin to feel deeply relaxed.

You begin to feel more and more limp.

Your muscles be come more and more heavy.

You sink deeper into relaxation, far away from the cares of the world.

Back

This time focus your attention on the back muscles that are below the shoulders.

Tense up your lower back by pressing your back against the chair, or just tightening up. Do this now.

Let the tension build.

Let the muscles get nice and hard.

And let go.

(continued)

TABLE 3.5   *(continued)*

Let the tension go.

Feelings of tightness melt and flow away.

Let yourself feel more relaxed.

Let feelings of tightness go.

Back (Repeat)

Once again, tighten up your back muscles, now.

Create a good feeling of tension.

Take care not to tense up too much.

And let go.

Let your muscles go limp.

Release the tension.

Your back becomes more and more relaxed.

Feel the sensations of relaxation.

[HALFWAY POINT]

Shoulders

This time focus on your shoulder muscles, now.

Squeeze your shoulders, now.

Create a nice good shrug.

Let the feelings of tightness grow.

And let go.
Let the tension flow out.

Let your tension begin to unwind.

Let the muscles begin to smooth out.

Let the muscles become more deeply relaxed.

Shoulders (Repeat)

Again, squeeze the shoulder muscles, now.

Let the muscles get nice and hard.

Let the feelings of tightness grow

TABLE 3.5 *(continued)*

And let go.

Let the muscles go limp.

There is nothing you have to do.

Let feelings of tension dissolve.

Back of Neck

Focus on the muscles in the back of the neck.

Gently tilt your head back and gently press the back of your head against your neck, now.

Tighten up the muscles.

Squeeze the muscles more and more.

And let go.

Let the muscles become more deeply relaxed.

Let your entire body become loose and limp.

Let yourself sink deeper and deeper into relaxation.

Let yourself forget the tensions and cares of the world.

Back of Neck (Repeat)

Once again, tighten up the back of the neck, now.

Tighter and tighter.

Tense up only the muscles of back of the neck.

And let go.

Let the tension flow away.

Your muscles feel relaxed and soothed.

As you sink far away from the cares of the world.

Face

This time focus on the muscles of your face.

Squeeze them altogether, now.

Squeeze your jaws, tongue, lip, nose, eyes, eyebrows, and forehead . . . all together. Squeeze your entire face together.

(continued)

TABLE 3.5 *(continued)*

Let the feelings of tightness grow.

And let go.

Feel calm and relaxed.

Let the tension smooth out.

Sink deeper and deeper into relaxation.

Let the muscles relax.

Face (Repeat)

Once again, tighten up the muscles of the face, now.

Take care not to tense up too much.

Tense up only the muscles of the face.

And let go.

Let the tension go.

Let the tension flow out.

Let tension smooth out.

Let yourself forget the tensions and cares of the world.

Front of Neck

Focus on the muscles of the neck.

Bow your head and gently press your chin down to your chest, now.

Tighten up the muscles.

Let the tension grow.

And let go.

Let tension begin to melt into liquid.

Let the rest of your body remain relaxed.

Let yourself sink deeper and deeper into relaxation.

Let your entire body become more relaxed.

Front of Neck (repeat)

Again, tighten up the front of the neck, now.

TABLE 3.5 *(continued)*

Hold the tension.

Create a good feeling of tension.

And let go.

Let the muscles become more deeply relaxed.

Let your muscles go limp.

Let the muscles begin to smooth out.

There is nothing you have to do.

Stomach and Chest

Focus on the muscles of your stomach and chest.

Tighten them up, now.

(Tense your stomach and chest in whatever way feels best . . . by pulling your stomach in . . . pushing it out . . . or tightening it up.)

Let the muscles get nice and hard.

And let go.

Feelings of tension dissolve.

Let yourself feel more detached.

More and more relaxed.

Far away from the cares of the world.

Stomach and Chest (Repeat)

Tighten up the stomach and chest again, now.

Squeeze the muscles more and more.

Take care not to tense up too much.

And let go.

Release the tension.

Sink into a deep state of relaxation.

Distant and far away from the cares of the world

Right Leg

Focus on the muscles in your right leg.

(continued)

TABLE 3.5   *(continued)*

Tense the muscles in the leg, now (push your leg against the leg or back of your chair . . . or press your leg tightly against the other leg).

Tighten up the muscles.

Let the tension grow.

And let go.

Relax.

Sink deeper into relaxation.

Your muscles become more and more heavy, as you sink deep into relaxation.

Right Leg (Repeat)

Again, tighten up the right leg, now.

Let the feelings of tightness grow.

Let the tension feel satisfying and complete.

And let go.

Let your entire body go completely limp.

Let your whole body relax.

As you forget the cares of the world.

Feeling far away and relaxed.

Left Leg

And tighten up the muscle of the left leg, now.

Tighten up the muscles.

Let the muscles get nice and hard.

And let go.

Release the tension.

Let your entire body go limp.

Let the tension flow out.

As you become more and more relaxed.

TABLE 3.5 *(continued)*

Left Leg (Repeat)

Once again, tighten up the left leg, now.

Squeeze the muscles more and more.

Create a good feeling of tension.

And let go.

There is nothing you have to do.

Let the rest of your body remain relaxed.

Sink deeper into relaxation.

Right Foot

Focus on your right foot.

Tense up the muscles of the right foot and toes, now (curl your toes into the floor while pushing down).

Tighten up the muscles, now.

Tense up only the muscles of right foot.

And let go.

Let the tension flow out.

And you become more completely relaxed.

Completely passive and indifferent.

Far away from the cares of the world.

Right Foot (Repeat)

Again, tighten up the right foot, now.

Let the feelings of tightness grow

Squeeze the muscles more and more.

And let go.

Let the muscles become deeply relaxed.

Tension unwinds.

Forget the tensions and cares of the world.

Distant, far away.

(continued)

TABLE 3.5 *(continued)*

Left Foot

And tighten up your left foot, now.

Tighten up those muscles.

Let the muscles get nice and hard.

And let go.

Let your body become completely limp.

Tension begins to melt into liquid.

Any remaining tension flows out of your muscles.

Sink deeper and deeper into relaxation.

Left Foot (Repeat)

Again, tighten up the left foot, now.

Let the tension grow.

And let go.

Let your muscles go limp.

Limp and loose.

Sink into a deep state of relaxation.

Far away from the cares of the world.

Indifferent to the world.

Review

Quietly attend to how you feel.

Your hands and arms.

If you feel any leftover tension in your hands and arms, just let go. Go limp.

Your back and shoulders.

If you feel any leftover tension in your back and shoulders, just let go. Go limp.

Sink deeper and deeper into relaxation.

Your shoulders and neck.

TABLE 3.5   *(continued)*

If you feel any leftover tension in your shoulders and neck, just let go. Go completely limp.

Relax more and more.

Far away from the cares of the world.

The muscles of your face.

If you feel any leftover tension in the muscles of your face, just let go. Go completely limp.

Sink into a state of deep relaxation, indifferent to the cares and concerns of the world.

The muscles of your legs and feet.

If you feel any leftover tension in your legs and feet, just let go. Go completely limp.

Distant and far away.

Deep into relaxation.

And your entire body.

Is there any part of your body where you feel even the slightest bit of tension?

Just let go. Go completely limp.

Sink deeper and deeper, far away into relaxation.

[PAUSE 10 SECONDS]

Gently let go of what you are attending to.

[PAUSE]

Slowly open your eyes.

[PAUSE]

We have completed our relaxation exercise.

APPROACH 2: AUTOGENIC TRAINING

Autogenic training (AT) is perhaps the most widely taught approach to professional relaxation in Europe. The fundamental strategy is to mentally repeat phrases or images suggestive of somatic relaxation. Elsewhere (Smith, 1987), I have suggested two levels of autogenic exercises. Level 1 targets the surface of the body, specifically, sensations associated with the skin and skeletal muscles ("warm and heavy," "tingling"). Level 2 targets internal organs, structures, and processes such as the solar plexus ("I feel a warm glow in my abdomen"), gastrointestinal system and digestion ("My stomach is calm"), the heart ("slow and even heartbeat"), and breathing ("It breathes me"). Generally, Level 2 exercises require more skill at focusing and passivity. In America, focus has been on "warmth-heaviness" suggestions and organ-specific formulas ("My heart is beating quietly and strongly").

In my clinical experience, AT (at least the beginning exercises), like PMR, may facilitate Sleepiness, Disengagement, and Physical Relaxation. Autogenic exercises require a degree of focusing ability and are perhaps less appropriate for clients who are easily distracted or who need a highly structured and familiar training format. Although proponents claim the approach can be applied to virtually any condition, a conservative strategy is to apply it in situations where autonomic arousal is clearly involved (see Table 3.7 at end of chapter) or to supplement or follow PMR.

One should seek medical approval before attempting autogenic suggestions for organs or processes that are weakened, injured, recovering from surgery, under treatment, or whose functioning is compromised in any way. For example, if a client suffers from abdominal bleeding, it would not be wise to suggest, "My stomach is warm and throbbing." Such a suggestion might conceivably increase blood flow to the abdomen. For a client suffering from cold hands, obviously do not suggest "My hands are cool and relaxed."

When presenting autogenic exercises, speak in a slow monotone. Voice quality for autogenic exercises should be similar to the PMR "let go" voice previously discussed. Speak in a slow and boring monotone, adding little color or interest to what you are saying.

Step 1: Explanation and Rationale

When presenting autogenic exercises, explain the key idea of the connection between body and mind. For example, imagining the taste of a lemon can often evoke the somatic response of salivation. Similarly, thoughts can evoke bodily relaxation. When we relax, we feel physical changes, for example, heaviness, warmth, an evenly beating heart, slow breathing. Autogenic exercises make use of these feelings. The technique is to simply and passively repeat phrases or images that suggest these relaxation feelings. If clients are given the full 6-week program, explain that each week they will add a technique. Starting with 2 minutes and going up to 10, at the end of the program clients will have a complete program of relaxation.

Step 2: Demonstration

First, demonstrate the importance of passive, as opposed to active thinking. Here is a demonstration I use (Smith, 1987):

> First, let's demonstrate its opposite, active thinking. Let your right hand drop to your side. Now, actively and effortfully try to make your hand feel warm and heavy. Work at it. Exert as much effort as you can trying to actively and deliberately will your hands to feel warm and heavy.
>
> Now, simply relax. Let your hand fall limply by your side. Without trying to accomplish anything, simply let the phrase "My hand is warm and heavy" repeat in your mind. Let the words repeat on their own, like an echo. All you have to do is quietly observe the repeating words. Don't try to achieve warmth and heaviness. Just quietly let the words go over and over in your mind. While thinking the words "warm and heavy," you might want to imagine your hand in warm sand, or in the sun, or in a warm bath. Pick an image that feels comfortable, and simple dwell upon it.
>
> We have just tried active and passive thinking. Which was more effective? (p. 134)

Explain each of the phrases that will be employed. The options include any combination of the following (Linden, 1993):

"Heavy." This suggestion is claimed to increase muscle relaxation. A relaxed muscle will actually feel "heavy," because less effort is exerted keeping the muscle firm. You may notice this when, after an exhausting day, you fall heavily into a bed. Or perhaps you become so relaxed in a chair that you can barely get up.

"Warm." This suggestion is claimed to increase blood flow to the fingers, hands, and feet. When relaxed, blood flow increases to the extremities, contributing to feelings of warmth. In contrast, when under stress, blood flows away from the extremities, contributing to "cold, clammy hands."

"Quiet, even beating heart." Most people understand that when under stress, the heart starts beating hard, sometimes irregularly. This suggestion fosters a relaxed heartbeat.

"It breathes me" or "My breathing is free and easy and effortless." When relaxed, breathing is more slow and even. Breathing is both voluntary and involuntary. We can deliberately take in a deep breath. But we continue breathing even when not thinking about it. In this exercise, we simply watch the process of passive, relaxed breathing. Linden uses the suggestion "It breathes me." In my experience, clients can find this concept troublesome; I prefer "My breathing is free and easy and effortless." I suggest omitting AT breathing exercises because they are redundant with formal breathing exercises presented elsewhere.

The following somewhat more advanced exercises are optional.

"Sun rays streaming warm and quiet." In this suggestion, one focuses on the solar plexus, an important nerve center for internal organs. The solar plexus is halfway between the navel and the lower portion of the sternum in the upper half of the body.

"The forehead is cool." This suggestion targets feelings one might have from placing a soothing, cool washcloth on the forehead. I suggest omitting this exercise for most clients because the resulting R-State is often Mental Relaxation and Strength and Awareness, rather than Disengagement and Physical Relaxation.

Other autogenic suggestions can be selected from words associated with the R-States Physical or Mental Relaxation ("I feel limp, loose, liquid" etc.). Linden (1993) suggests that personalized suggestions be positive ("I feel more calm" vs. "I feel less tense"). Also, they should be consistent with a client's beliefs. Finally, suggestions should be phrased in a way that is pleasing and simple to recite or think. For example, one might employ simple words, rhymes, and internal rhythms. A useful insomnia suggestion might be "My sleep is deep and peaceful" rather than "I will fall asleep more quickly tonight."

Step 3: Dress Rehearsal

Dress rehearsal sessions can last from 2 to 9 minutes, depending on how many suggestion combinations are included. For the full program described by Linden (1993), one technique is added a week, using a schedule similar to this. See Table 3.8 for a complete autogenic training script.

Week 1:

"Arms and legs are heavy" (2 min).

Week 2:

"Arms and legs are heavy" (2 min).

"Arms and legs are very warm" (2 min).

Week 3:

"Arms and legs are heavy" (1 min).

"Arms and legs are very warm" (1 min).

"Heart is beating quietly and strongly" (2 min).

Week 4 (can be used for one-session presentation):

"Arms and legs are heavy" (1 min).

"Arms and legs are very warm" (1 min).

"Heart is beating quietly and strongly" (2 min).

"My breathing is free and easy and effortless" (2 min; optional).

(The following weeks are optional.)

Week 5:

"Arms and legs are heavy" (1 min).

"Arms and legs are very warm" (1 min).

"Heart is beating quietly and strongly" (1 min).

"My breathing is free and easy and effortless" (2 min).

"Sun rays are streaming quiet and warm." (2 min).

Week 6:

"Arms and legs are heavy" (1 min).

"Arms and legs are very warm" (1 min).

"Heart is beating quietly and strongly" (1 min).

"My breathing is free and easy and effortless" (2 min).

"Sun rays are streaming quiet and warm" (2 min).

"The forehead is cool" (2 min).

Steps 4 and 5: Checking and Modification

Check for problems that arise. Cease techniques that cause any difficulty or frustration.

The following are suggestions for enhancing AT:

• Precede or integrate PMR exercises that, like AT, tend to evoke the R-States Physical Relaxation and Disengagement.
• Incorporate imagery suggestive of targeted physical processes ("Imagine you are on the beach, enjoying the warm sand, sun, and water").
• Passive breathing exercises may be introduced.
• Avoid yoga stretching or active breathing exercises.
• Avoid active narrative or insight imagery, as these can evoke R-States inconsistent with AT.
• For some clients it may be appropriate to end with a simple meditation, given that this technique can cultivate disengagement.
• Supplement with casual relaxation activities that might also foster Physical Relaxation, Disengagement, and possibly Sleepiness. These include hot baths, sun bathing, and massage.
• Select a soothing and unstimulating practice environment conducive to Sleepiness and Disengagement.

TABLE 3.8   Six-Week Sequence of Autogenic Exercises

(Words that are in **boldface** or [BRACKETED] are special instructions to trainers. These words are not to be read or spoken to clients.)

WEEK 1   [CAN BE PRESENTED ALONE]

Heavy

Let yourself sink into a comfortable state of relaxation, far away from the cares of the world. This time is just for you; you can forget the problems of the day.

TABLE 3.8 *(continued)*

Quietly attend to your right arm.

[PAUSE]

Simply think the words, "The right (or dominant) hand is very heavy. Very heavy. Very heavy."

[PAUSE]

There is no need for you to achieve any effect.

[PAUSE]

Like there is a weight, a heavy book, softly resting on your right arm. Or like a magnet pulling tension away. Making it more and more heavy.

[PAUSE]

Right hand is very heavy. Very heavy.

[PAUSE]

Right hand is very heavy. Very heavy.

[PAUSE 5 SECONDS]

Let yourself sink into a distant state of pleasant relaxation.

[PAUSE 5 SECONDS]

Calm and relaxed.

[PAUSE]

Very quiet.

[PAUSE]

There is nothing you have to do.

[PAUSE]

Let the words go over and over like an echo.

[PAUSE]

(continued)

TABLE 3.8 *(continued)*

Right arm is very heavy. Very heavy. Very heavy.

[PAUSE 5 SECONDS]

There is nothing you have to do.

[PAUSE 5 SECONDS]

Let tension sink away.

[PAUSE 5 SECONDS]

Let gravity pull tension away.

[PAUSE]

As you forget your cares and concerns.

[PAUSE]

The right arm is very heavy. Very heavy. Very heavy.

[PAUSE 5 SECONDS]

Your arm becomes more and more loose and limp.

[PAUSE]

As tension sinks away.

[PAUSE]

Like a magnet pulling tension away.

[PAUSE 5 SECONDS]

You become more calm and relaxed, very quiet.

[PAUSE 5 SECONDS]

The right arm is very heavy.

[PAUSE 5 SECONDS]

The right arm is very heavy.

[PAUSE 5 SECONDS]

The right arm is very heavy.

Let yourself sink into a distant state of pleasant relaxation.

TABLE 3.8   *(continued)*

[PAUSE 5 SECONDS]

   Calm and relaxed.

[PAUSE]

   Very quiet.

[PAUSE]

   There is nothing you have to do.

[PAUSE]

   Let the words, go over and over like an echo.

[PAUSE]

   Left arm is very heavy. Very heavy. Very heavy.

[PAUSE 5 SECONDS]

   There is nothing you have to do.

[PAUSE 5 SECONDS]

   Let tension sink away.

[PAUSE 5 SECONDS]

   Let gravity pull tension away.

[PAUSE]

   As you forget your cares and concerns

[PAUSE]

   The left arm is very heavy. Very heavy. Very heavy.

[PAUSE 5 SECONDS]

   Your arm becomes more and more loose and limp.

[PAUSE]

   As tension sinks away.

[PAUSE]

(continued)

TABLE 3.8 *(continued)*

Like a magnet pulling tension away.

[PAUSE 5 SECONDS]

You become more calm and relaxed, very quiet.

[PAUSE 5 SECONDS]

The left arm is very heavy.

[PAUSE 5 SECONDS]

The left arm is very heavy.

[PAUSE 5 SECONDS]

The left arm is very heavy.

[PAUSE 10 SECONDS]

WEEK 2

Heavy

let yourself sink into a comfortable state of relaxation, far away from the cares of the world. This time is just for you; you can forget the problems of the day.

Simply think the words "Arms and legs are very heavy."

[PAUSE]

There is no need for you to achieve any effect.

[PAUSE]

Arms and legs are very heavy, like gravity is pulling them toward the earth.

Like a magnet is pulling tension away.

[PAUSE 5 SECONDS]

Arms and legs more and more heavy.

TABLE 3.8 *(continued)*

[PAUSE 5 SECONDS]

Let yourself sink into a distant state of pleasant relaxation.

[PAUSE]

There is nothing you have to do.

[PAUSE]

Let the words go over and over like an echo.

[PAUSE]

Arms and legs very heavy. Very heavy. Very heavy.

[PAUSE]

There is nothing you have to do.

[PAUSE]

Let tension sink away.

[PAUSE]

Let gravity pull tension away.

[PAUSE]

As you forget your cares and concerns.

[PAUSE]

You become more calm and relaxed.

[PAUSE]

More quiet.

[PAUSE 5 SECONDS]

Your arms and legs are very heavy.

[PAUSE]

Very heavy.

[PAUSE]

(continued)

TABLE 3.8 *(continued)*

Very heavy.

[PAUSE 5 SECONDS]

Your arms becomes more and more loose and limp.

[PAUSE]

As tension sinks away.

[PAUSE]

Like a magnet pulling tension away.

[PAUSE]

Arms and legs are very heavy.

[PAUSE]

Arms and legs are very heavy.

[PAUSE]

Arms and legs are very heavy.

[PAUSE 5 SECONDS]

Warm

The right (dominant) arm is heavy and warm.

[PAUSE]

Arm is heavy, arm is warm.

[PAUSE]

Like the warm sun is shining on the arm.

[PAUSE]

Dissolving feelings of tension.

[PAUSE]

Tension melts and flows away.

TABLE 3.8 *(continued)*

[PAUSE]

Arm is heavy and warm.

[PAUSE]

Like warm water is flowing on the arm.

[PAUSE]

Dissolving feelings of tension.

[PAUSE 5 SECONDS]

Tension melts and flows away.

[PAUSE 5 SECONDS]

Arm is warm.

[PAUSE]

Arm is warm and relaxed.

[PAUSE]

Let yourself sink deeper into a pleasant state of relaxation.

[PAUSE]

Relaxed and calm.

[PAUSE 5 SECONDS]

Far away from the cares of the world.

[PAUSE 5 SECONDS]

Far away.

[PAUSE 5 SECONDS]

Warm and heavy.

[PAUSE]

Sink into deeper relaxation, heavy and warm.

(continued)

TABLE 3.8   *(continued)*

The left arm is heavy and warm.

[PAUSE]

Arm is heavy, arm is warm.

[PAUSE]

Like the warm sun is shining on the arm.

[PAUSE]

Dissolving feelings of tension.

[PAUSE]

Tension melts and flows away.

[PAUSE]

Arm is heavy and warm.

[PAUSE]

Like warm water is flowing on the arm.

[PAUSE]

Dissolving feelings of tension.

[PAUSE 5 SECONDS]

Tension melts and flows away.

[PAUSE 5 SECONDS]

Arm is warm.

[PAUSE]

Arm is warm and relaxed.

[PAUSE]

Let yourself sink deeper into a pleasant state of relaxation.

[PAUSE]

Relaxed and calm.

[PAUSE 5 SECONDS]

TABLE 3.8 *(continued)*

Far away from the cares of the world.

[PAUSE 5 SECONDS]

Far away.

[PAUSE 5 SECONDS]

Warm and heavy.

[PAUSE]

Sink into deeper relaxation, heavy and warm.

[PAUSE]

WEEK 3

Heavy

Let yourself sink into a comfortable state of relaxation, far away from the cares of the world. This time is just for you; you can forget the problems of the day.

[PAUSE 5 SECONDS]

Simply think the words, "Arms and legs are very heavy."

[PAUSE 5 SECONDS]

There is no need for you to achieve any effect.

[PAUSE 5 SECONDS]

Arms and legs are very heavy, like gravity is pulling them toward the earth. Like a magnet is pulling tension away.

[PAUSE 5 SECONDS]

Arms and legs more and more heavy.

[PAUSE 5 SECONDS]

Let yourself sink into a distant state of pleasant relaxation.

(continued)

TABLE 3.8   *(continued)*

[PAUSE 5 SECONDS]

   There is nothing you have to do.

[PAUSE 5 SECONDS]

   Let the words go over and over like an echo.

[PAUSE]

   Arms and legs very heavy. Very heavy. Very heavy.

[PAUSE]

   There is nothing you have to do.

[PAUSE]

   Let tension sink away.

[PAUSE]

   Let gravity pull tension away.

[PAUSE]

   As you forget your cares and concerns

[PAUSE 5 SECONDS]

   You become more calm and relaxed.

[PAUSE]

   More quiet.

[PAUSE]

   Your arms and legs are very heavy. Very heavy. Very heavy.

[PAUSE]

   Your arm becomes more and more loose and limp.

[PAUSE]

   As tension sinks away.

[PAUSE 5 SECONDS]

TABLE 3.8   *(continued)*

Like a magnet pulling tension away.

[PAUSE]

Arms and legs are very heavy.

[PAUSE]

Arms and legs are very heavy.

[PAUSE]

Arms and legs are very heavy.

[PAUSE]

Warm

Arms and legs are heavy and warm.

[PAUSE]

Arms and legs are warm.

[PAUSE]

Like the warm sun is shining.

[PAUSE]

Dissolving feelings of tension.

[PAUSE]

Tension melts and flows away.

[PAUSE]

Arms and legs are heavy and warm.

[PAUSE 5 SECONDS]

Like warm water is flowing on your body.

[PAUSE]

Dissolving feelings of tension.

[PAUSE]

(continued)

TABLE 3.8 *(continued)*

Tension melts and flows away.

[PAUSE]

Arms and legs are warm.

[PAUSE]

Warm and relaxed.

[PAUSE]

Let yourself sink deeper into a pleasant state of relaxation.

[PAUSE]

Relaxed and calm.

[PAUSE]

Far away from the cares of the world.

[PAUSE]

Far away.

[PAUSE 5 SECONDS]

Warm and heavy.

[PAUSE]

Sink into deeper relaxation, heavy and warm.

Heart

Gently rest your hand on your chest, over your heart.

[PAUSE]

Think the words "Heart is beating quietly and strongly, quietly and evenly."

[PAUSE]

TABLE 3.8   *(continued)*

Heart is beating quietly and evenly.

[PAUSE]

As your body sinks deeper into comfortable relaxation.

[PAUSE]

Far away from the cares of the world.

[PAUSE]

Heart is warm, beating quietly and evenly.

[PAUSE]

Quietly and evenly.

[PAUSE 5 SECONDS]

As gravity pulls tension from your body.

[PAUSE]

As the warm sun melts tension from your body.

[PAUSE]

You settle into a safe and comfortable relaxation

[PAUSE]

Heart is beating, quietly and evenly.

[PAUSE]

Quietly and evenly.

[PAUSE]

There is nothing you have to do.

[PAUSE 5 SECONDS]

As you become more comfortably relaxed.

[PAUSE]

WEEK 4/ALTERNATIVE SINGLE-SESSION PRESENTATION

Let yourself sink into a comfortable state of relaxation, far away

---

(continued)

TABLE 3.8 *(continued)*

from the cares of the world. This time is just for you; you can forget the problems of the day.

Heavy

Simply think the words "Hands and arms, very heavy."

There is no need for you to achieve any effect.

[PAUSE 5 SECONDS]

Hands and arms are very heavy, like gravity is pulling them toward the earth.

[PAUSE 5 SECONDS]

Like a magnet is pulling tension away.

[PAUSE 5 SECONDS]

Arms and legs getting heavy.

[PAUSE 5 SECONDS]

Gravity pulling them down.

[PAUSE 5 SECONDS]

Feel the heavy weight as your arms and legs sink.

[PAUSE 5 SECONDS]

Heavier and heavier.

[PAUSE 5 SECONDS]

Entire body, more and more heavy.

[PAUSE]

Let yourself sink into a distant state of pleasant relaxation.

[PAUSE]

There is nothing you have to do.

[PAUSE 5 SECONDS]

Let the words go over and over like an echo.

TABLE 3.8   *(continued)*

[PAUSE]

Arms and legs very heavy. Very heavy. Very heavy.

[PAUSE]

There is nothing you have to do.

[PAUSE]

Let tension sink away.

[PAUSE]

Let gravity pull tension away.

[PAUSE]

As you forget your cares and concerns

[PAUSE]

You become more calm and relaxed.

[PAUSE]

More quiet.

[PAUSE]

Entire body, very heavy. Very heavy. Very heavy.

[PAUSE 5 SECONDS]

Your arms become more and more loose and limp.

[PAUSE]

As tension sinks away.

[PAUSE]

Like a magnet pulling tension away.

[PAUSE]

Arms and legs are very heavy.

[PAUSE]

(continued)

TABLE 3.8   *(continued)*

Entire body very heavy.

[PAUSE]

Arms and legs are very heavy.

[PAUSE 5 SECONDS]

Warm

Arms and legs are heavy and warm.

[PAUSE 5 SECONDS]

Entire body, nice and warm.

[PAUSE 5 SECONDS]

Like the warm sun is shining.

[PAUSE]

Dissolving feelings of tension.

[PAUSE]

Tension melts and flows away.

[PAUSE]

Arms and legs are heavy and warm.

[PAUSE]

Like warm water is flowing on your body.

[PAUSE 5 SECONDS]

Dissolving feelings of tension.

[PAUSE]

Tension melts and flows away.

[PAUSE]

Entire body very warm

TABLE 3.8 *(continued)*

[PAUSE]

Warm and relaxed.

[PAUSE 5 SECONDS]

Let yourself sink deeper into a pleasant state of relaxation.

[PAUSE]

Relaxed and calm.

[PAUSE]

Far away from the cares of the world.

[PAUSE 5 SECONDS]

Far away.

[PAUSE 5 SECONDS]

Warm and heavy.

[PAUSE 5 SECONDS]

Sink into deeper relaxation, heavy and warm.

Heart

Think the words "Heart is beating quietly and strongly, quietly and evenly."

[PAUSE 5 SECONDS]

Heart is beating quietly and evenly.

[PAUSE 5 SECONDS]

As your body sinks deeper into comfortable relaxation.

[PAUSE 5 SECONDS]

Far away from the cares of the world.

[PAUSE 5 SECONDS]

(continued)

TABLE 3.8 *(continued)*

Heart is warm, beating quietly and evenly.

[PAUSE]

Quietly and evenly.

[PAUSE]

As gravity pulls tension from your body.

[PAUSE 5 SECONDS]

As the warm sun melts tension from your body.

[PAUSE 5 SECONDS]

You settle into a safe and comfortable relaxation

[PAUSE]

Heart is beating, quietly and evenly.

[PAUSE 5 SECONDS]

Quietly and evenly.

[PAUSE]

There is nothing you have to do.

[PAUSE]

As you become more comfortably relaxed.

WEEK 5

Let yourself sink into a comfortable state of relaxation, far away from the cares of the world. This time is just for you; you can forget the problems of the day.

[PAUSE 5 SECONDS]

Heavy

Simply think the words, "Whole body, very heavy." There is no need for you to achieve any effect.

TABLE 3.8   *(continued)*

[PAUSE]

Arms and legs are very heavy, like gravity is pulling them toward the earth. Like a magnet is pulling tension away.

[PAUSE]

Entire body, more and more heavy.

[PAUSE]

Let yourself sink into a distant state of pleasant relaxation.

[PAUSE]

There is nothing you have to do.

[PAUSE]

Let the words go over and over like an echo.

[PAUSE]

Arms and legs very heavy. Very heavy. Very heavy.

[PAUSE]

There is nothing you have to do.

[PAUSE]

Let tension sink away.

[PAUSE]

Let gravity pull tension away.

[PAUSE]

As you forget your cares and concerns

[PAUSE 5 SECONDS]

You become more calm and relaxed.

[PAUSE]

(continued)

TABLE 3.8   *(continued)*

More quiet.

[PAUSE 5 SECONDS]

Entire body, very heavy. Very heavy. Very heavy.

[PAUSE 5 SECONDS]

Your arms become more and more loose and limp.

[PAUSE]

As tension sinks away.

[PAUSE]

Like a magnet pulling tension away.

[PAUSE 5 SECONDS]

Arms and legs are very heavy.

[PAUSE]

Entire body very heavy.

[PAUSE]

Arms and legs are very heavy.

[PAUSE]

Warm

Arms and legs are heavy and warm.

[PAUSE 5 SECONDS]

Entire body, nice and warm.

[PAUSE]

Like the warm sun is shining.

[PAUSE]

Dissolving feelings of tension.

[PAUSE]

TABLE 3.8   *(continued)*

Tension melts and flows away.

[PAUSE]

Arms and legs are heavy and warm.

[PAUSE 5 SECONDS]

Like warm water is flowing on your body.

[PAUSE]

Dissolving feelings of tension.

[PAUSE]

Tension melts and flows away.

[PAUSE]

Entire body very warm

[PAUSE]

Warm and relaxed.

[PAUSE]

Let yourself sink deeper into a pleasant state of relaxation.

[PAUSE 5 SECONDS]

Relaxed and calm.

[PAUSE 5 SECONDS]

Far away from the cares of the world.

[PAUSE 5 SECONDS]

Far away.

[PAUSE]

Warm and heavy.

[PAUSE]

(continued)

TABLE 3.8 *(continued)*

Sink into deeper relaxation, heavy and warm.

[PAUSE]

Heart

[PAUSE 5 SECONDS]

Think the words "Heart is beating quietly and strongly, quietly and evenly."

[PAUSE 5 SECONDS]

Heart is beating quietly and evenly.

[PAUSE 5 SECONDS]

As your body sinks deeper into comfortable relaxation.

[PAUSE]

Far away from the cares of the world.

[PAUSE]

Heart is warm, beating quietly and evenly.

[PAUSE]

Quietly and evenly.

[PAUSE]

As gravity pulls tension from your body.

[PAUSE 5 SECONDS]

As the warm sun melts tension from your body.

[PAUSE 5 SECONDS]

You settle into a safe and comfortable relaxation

[PAUSE 5 SECONDS]

Heart is beating quietly and evenly.

[PAUSE 5 SECONDS]

TABLE 3.8   *(continued)*

Quietly and evenly.

[PAUSE 5 SECONDS]

There is nothing you have to do.

[PAUSE 5 SECONDS]

As you become more comfortably relaxed.

[PAUSE 5 SECONDS]

Your breathing becomes even and relaxed.

[PAUSE 5 SECONDS]

There is no reason to try to breathe in any way.

[PAUSE 5 SECONDS]

Let your body breathe on its own.

[PAUSE 5 SECONDS]

Think the words "My breathing is free and easy and effortless; it breathes me." There is no need to create any change. Just think the words, like an echo. Over and over.

[PAUSE 5 SECONDS]

My breathing is free and easy and effortless.

[PAUSE 5 SECONDS]

With every breath, sink deeper and deeper into relaxation.

[PAUSE 5 SECONDS]

My breathing is free and easy and effortless.

[PAUSE 5 SECONDS]

Far away from the cares of the world.

[PAUSE 5 SECONDS]

My breathing is free and easy and effortless.

(continued)

TABLE 3.8 *(continued)*

[PAUSE 5 SECONDS]

Solar Plexus

And now gently attend to an area above your navel.

[PAUSE]

An area where you feel warm and good after drinking warm hot chocolate or good soup.

Imagine sun rays streaming from this area, quiet and warm.

[PAUSE]

Warming your abdomen.

[PAUSE]

Warming and relaxing your entire inside.

[PAUSE]

Sun rays streaming quiet and warm.

[PAUSE]

Let yourself sink deeper into relaxation.

[PAUSE]

Far away from the cares of the world.

[PAUSE]

Imagine sun rays streaming quiet and warm.

[PAUSE]

Let yourself become more and more deeply relaxed.

[PAUSE 5 SECONDS]

More and more quiet and calm.

TABLE 3.8 *(continued)*

[PAUSE 5 SECONDS]

Soothing away the tensions of the day.

[PAUSE 5 SECONDS]

Sun rays streaming quiet and warm.

[PAUSE]

Sun rays streaming quiet and warm.

[PAUSE 5 SECONDS]

WEEK 6

Let yourself sink into a comfortable state of relaxation, far away from the cares of the world. This time is just for you; you can forget the problems of the day.

[PAUSE]

Heavy

Simply think the words "Hands and arms, very heavy."

[PAUSE]

There is no need for you to achieve any effect.

[PAUSE]

Arms and legs growing heavy, like gravity is pulling them toward the earth. Like a magnet is pulling tension away.

[PAUSE]

Hands and arms, growing heavy.

Arms and legs, growing heavy.

Entire body, more and more heavy.

[PAUSE]

Let yourself sink into a distant state of pleasant relaxation.

(continued)

TABLE 3.8 *(continued)*

[PAUSE]

There is nothing you have to do.

[PAUSE]

Let the words, go over and over like an echo.

[PAUSE]

Arms and legs very heavy. Very heavy. Very heavy.

[PAUSE]

There is nothing you have to do.

[PAUSE]

Let tension sink away.

[PAUSE]

Let gravity pull tension away.

[PAUSE]

As you forget your cares and concerns

[PAUSE]

You become more calm and relaxed.

[PAUSE]

More quiet.

[PAUSE]

Entire body, very heavy. Very heavy. Very heavy.

[PAUSE]

Your arms become more and more loose and limp.

[PAUSE]

TABLE 3.8   *(continued)*

As tension sinks away.

[PAUSE]

Like a magnet pulling tension away.

[PAUSE]

Arms and legs are very heavy.

[PAUSE]

Entire body very heavy.

[PAUSE]

Arms and legs are very heavy.

Warm

Arms and legs are heavy and warm.

[PAUSE]

Entire body, nice and warm.

[PAUSE]

Like the warm sun is shining.

[PAUSE]

Dissolving feelings of tension.

[PAUSE]

Tension melts and flows away.

[PAUSE]

Arms and legs are heavy and warm.

[PAUSE 5 SECONDS]

Like warm water is flowing on your body.

[PAUSE]

(continued)

TABLE 3.8 *(continued)*

Dissolving feelings of tension.

[PAUSE]

Tension melts and flows away.

[PAUSE]

Entire body very warm.

[PAUSE]

Warm and relaxed.

[PAUSE]

Let yourself sink deeper into a pleasant state of relaxation.

[PAUSE]

Relaxed and calm.

[PAUSE]

Far away from the cares of the world.

[PAUSE]

Far away.

[PAUSE 5 SECONDS]

Warm and heavy.

[PAUSE 5 SECONDS]

Sink into deeper relaxation, heavy and warm.

[PAUSE 5 SECONDS]

Heart

Think the words "Heart is beating quietly and strongly, heart is beating quietly and evenly."

[PAUSE]

Heart is beating quietly, strongly, quietly and evenly.

TABLE 3.8   *(continued)*

[PAUSE]

   As your body sinks deeper into comfortable relaxation.

[PAUSE]

   Far away from the cares of the world.

[PAUSE 5 SECONDS]

   Heart is warm, beating quietly, strongly.

[PAUSE 5 SECONDS]

   Quietly and evenly.

[PAUSE]

   As gravity pulls tension from your body.

[PAUSE]

   As the warm sun melts tension from your body.

[PAUSE 5 SECONDS]

   You settle into a safe and comfortable relaxation.

[PAUSE 5 SECONDS]

   Heart is beating quietly and evenly.

[PAUSE]

   Quietly and evenly.

[PAUSE]

   There is nothing you have to do.

[PAUSE]

   As you become more comfortably relaxed.

Breathing

   Your breathing becomes even and relaxed.

(continued)

TABLE 3.8 *(continued)*

[PAUSE]

There is no reason to try to breathe in any way.

[PAUSE]

Let your body breathe on its own.

[PAUSE]

Think the words "My breathing is free and easy and effortless; it breathes me."

[PAUSE 5 SECONDS]

There is no need to create any change.

[PAUSE]

Just think the words, like an echo. Over and over

[PAUSE 5 SECONDS]

My breathing is free and easy and effortless.

[PAUSE 5 SECONDS]

With every breath, sink deeper and deeper into relaxation.

[PAUSE 5 SECONDS]

My breathing is free and easy and effortless.

[PAUSE 5 SECONDS]

Far away from the cares of the world.

[PAUSE]

My breathing is free and easy and effortless.

Solar Plexus

And now gently attend to an area above your navel.

[PAUSE]

TABLE 3.8   *(continued)*

An area where you feel warm and good after drinking warm hot chocolate or good soup.

[PAUSE]

Imagine sun rays streaming from this area, quiet and warm.

[PAUSE]

Warming your abdomen.

[PAUSE]

Warming and relaxing your entire inside.

[PAUSE]

Sun rays streaming quiet and warm.

[PAUSE]

Let yourself sink deeper into relaxation.

[PAUSE]

Far away from the cares of the world.

[PAUSE]

Imagine sun rays streaming quiet and warm.

[PAUSE]

Let yourself become more and more deeply relaxed.

[PAUSE]

More and more quiet and calm.

[PAUSE 5 SECONDS]

Soothing away the tensions of the day.

[PAUSE 5 SECONDS]

Sun rays streaming quiet and warm.

(continued)

TABLE 3.8   *(continued)*

[PAUSE 5 SECONDS]

Sun rays streaming quiet and warm.

Forehead

Now focus on your forehead.

[PAUSE 5 SECONDS]

Think the words "Forehead is cool, forehead cool."

[PAUSE 5 SECONDS]

Like a cool moist cloth on your forehead.

[PAUSE 5 SECONDS]

Sink deeper into relaxation, far away from the cares of the world.

[PAUSE 5 SECONDS]

Forehead cool and relaxed.

[PAUSE 5 SECONDS]

Deeper into relaxation.

[PAUSE 5 SECONDS]

Forehead cool and relaxed.

[PAUSE 5 SECONDS]

And gently let go of what you are attending to.

[PAUSE]

Slowly open your eyes.

[PAUSE]

We have completed our relaxation exercise.

APPROACH 3: BREATHING

Breathing exercises are almost always deployed as a part of another technique. Traditional approaches include Lamaze, the natural childbirth method, and prana yoga. Breathing exercises vary considerably and include active yoga stretches, active diaphragmatic breathing, and passive approaches. Generally, the goal of breathing exercises is to foster diaphragmatic breathing and a pace that is slow, deep, and even. Relatively little research has examined the impact of breathing exercises. In our own research, we have found a strong connection between yoga breathing exercises and the R-States Mental Relaxation and Strength and Awareness. In contrast, autogenic breathing suggestions ("My breathing is free and easy and effortless") and variations of Van Dixhoorn's (1994) "breathing awareness" technique ("do the technique in a 'lazy,' or indifferent, almost careless way," without conscious effort to breathe in any particular way) may foster Disengagement. One can speculate that breathing relaxation might contribute to rapid reductions in affective arousal (Fried, 1993). See Table 3.9 at end of chapter.

Breathing exercises may not be appropriate for clients with temporal lobe epilepsy or those who suffer from psychosis (Fried, 1993). Active and diaphragmatic breathing exercises should be avoided by clients who have any abdominal injury or weakness or are recovering from abdominal surgery. Such techniques may also contribute to rapid blood oxygenation, an abrupt change that could be stressful for cardiac patients.

A special voice quality is appropriate for breathing exercises. Pattern instructions to follow your own inhalations and exhalations; that is, as you instruct a client to "inhale," inhale yourself. As you instruct a client to "exhale," breathe out. In addition, add a touch of "breathiness" to your speech, increasing the flow of air as you speak each word. Your voice should not convey the slow monotony of PMR and AT. Instead, cultivate a voice that sounds refreshed, relaxed, and alert.

Step 1: Explanation and Rationale

Explain that the way we breathe reflects our level of tension and relaxation. We breathe quickly and choppily when angry, momentarily hold our breath when afraid, gasp when shocked, and choke when in despair. In contrast, we sigh deeply when relieved. When we are deeply relaxed, our breathing is full, even, and unhurried.

To understand breathing and relaxation, clients need to understand something about the process of respiration. We breathe, of course, through the lungs. However, the lungs do not do the work of drawing in and expelling air. This is accomplished by the surrounding rib cage and collarbone, and by the diaphragm, an important drumlike muscle under the lungs that separates the chest cavity from the stomach.

Tense breathing is most likely to incorporate the rib cage and collarbone. Note that this can be seen in boxers or joggers, people who in their sport are necessarily quite tense in readiness. These people breathe "through the chest," and their shoulders may even rise and fall with every breath. Of course, such chest and collarbone movement helps breathing somewhat, by pulling the lungs open so that air can be drawn in.

Relaxed breathing begins with the diaphragm. When we inhale, the diaphragm pulls down, like a piston, and out, and the lungs expand with air. When we exhale, the diaphragm muscles relax inward and move up, forcing air out. Such diaphragmatic breathing is generally more easy and efficient than chest breathing. There are simply more blood vessels in the lower part of the lungs, near the diaphragm. Also, diaphragmatic breathing uses the least amount of energy to accomplish the work of breathing.

Here is a simple demonstration of the efficiency and ease of diaphragmatic breathing (Smith, 1989).

> First sit up comfortably with your feet flat on the floor. Place your hands gently over your stomach, so your thumbs are below your lowest rib. Now, breathe in through your chest. Keep your stomach as still as possible. Breathe in and out only through your chest. [PAUSE FOR 3 OR 4 INHALATIONS.] Now relax. This time we will breathe in a different way. Keep your hands over your stomach. When breathing in, hold your ribcage and collarbone as still as possible and breathe in through your stomach as slowly as you can. Imagine you are filling your stomach with air. Can you feel your stomach move as you inhale? Breathe in and out this way for about a minute or so. [PAUSE FOR 3 OR 4 INHALATIONS.]
>
> Most people find they can breathe more slowly and with less strain "through the stomach" than "through the chest." This is because stomach breathing involves primarily the diaphragm and is more efficient. (p. 114)

Relaxed breathing has a special rhythm. Exhalation is slow, even, and relatively passive. Muscle tension generated through inhalation is "let go" or "given up." The chest muscles and diaphragm relax automatically while air is quietly expelled. Although air is flowing through the lungs and out, there is a sinking movement associated with the automatic relaxation of the breathing muscles. When air has been exhaled, there is a pause until the need for oxygen prompts an automatic and relaxed inhalation. The inhalation phase occurs quietly and easily. In contrast, the rhythm of tense breathing is more active and forced. Inhalation is more effortful and pronounced. The breath is retained too long, until tension or discomfort forces a rapid exhalation.

The breathing exercises in this program are designed to encourage relaxed, full, and rhythmical breathing as well as to increase the ability to detect and differentiate between relaxed and tense breathing. They are meant to help one breathe diaphragmatically, deeply, evenly, and slowly.

Step 2: Demonstration

Clients can try three types of breathing exercises: active breathing stretches, active diaphragmatic breathing, and passive breathing. See Table 3.10 for verbatim instructions.

Active breathing stretches are designed to deliberately but somewhat indirectly foster diaphragmatic and slow breathing. Exercises include body arch breathing, bowing and breathing, bowing and stretching.

The general idea of these exercises is to exhale while bowing and inhale while stretching. Such pacing automatically fosters appropriate movement of the diaphragm. Beginning instructors can have difficulty timing the pace of stretching, bowing, and breathing. It can be useful to keep several points in mind. Observe the client. Look for nonverbal clues that a client is ready to inhale, and then suggest inhaling. When a client is ready to exhale, suggest exhaling. Even though exhaling should be associated with bowing, inhaling with stretching, clients will obviously have to breathe both in and out while bowing and stretching. When a client has to inhale during bowing, simply suggest that "it is OK to pause and take a breath." When exhaling during stretching, suggest that "it is OK to pause and exhale." Then continue. This enables a client to breathe naturally, without anxiety, and to emphasize exhaling during bowing, inhaling during stretching.

Active diaphragmatic breathing exercises also deliberately foster diaphragmatic breathing. These include stomach squeeze diaphragmatic breathing, stomach touch diaphragmatic breathing, and book breathing.

Passive breathing exercises foster a relaxed breathing pattern that is slow, even, and full. They include inhaling through nose, exhaling through lips, deep breathing, and focused breathing.

You may present all exercises in sequence or select those that appear most appropriate.

Step 3: Dress Rehearsal

Read or present a tape of selected exercises.

Steps 4 and 5: Checking and Modification

The active diaphragmatic exercises are most likely to present problems. From 5% to 15% of clients may display "paradoxical breathing," a pattern that involves extending the stomach (diaphragm down) while *exhaling* and pulling the stomach in (diaphragm up) while *inhaling*. To clients, this may seem natural, perhaps because the chest also extends out while breathing in. However, explain that this goes against the pattern of relaxed breathing; extending the stomach out should help inhalation, rather than exhalation. It is useful to illustrate this with a diagram. Clients may need to experiment with "book breathing" (resting a book over the abdomen and observing its movement during breathing) to discover how to pull the stomach in while exhaling.

A second problem some clients may have is anxiety and self-consciousness during breathing. Directing attention to the very process of inhaling and exhaling air can prove troublesome. Most clients adapt to this discomfort and can proceed with little additional concern. For clients who remain anxiously self-conscious about breathing, try presenting the active breathing stretches, deleting all references to breath, inhalation, exhalation, and air. The stretches, when done alone, can foster a relaxed and diaphragmatic pattern of breathing, even when breathing is not mentioned. If the problem continues, simply discontinue breathing exercises and try something else.

Some clients may experience signs of excessive oxygenation, including dizziness, faintness, and nausea. Shorten the exercise sequence or discontinue the exercise.

The following are suggestions for enhancing breathing exercises:

- Incorporate PMR tensing up with inhaling; exhale while letting go.
- Incorporate yogaform stretches.
- Incorporate imagery suggesting the relaxing flow of breath, wind, or air.
- End with meditation.

- Supplement with casual relaxation activities consistent with the desired target R-State. If Disengagement and Sleepiness are desired, consider autogenic type exercises. If Strength and Awareness is desired, consider imagery and yoga stretching.
- Practice in a setting conducive to feelings of Strength and Awareness.

TABLE 3.10   Breathing Relaxation Script

(Words that are in **boldface** or [BRACKETED] are special instructions to trainers. These words are not to be read or spoken to clients.)

ACTIVE BREATHING STRETCHES

Body Arch Breathing

Begin by making sure you are seated in an upright position.

[PAUSE]

Let the tensions of the day flow away.

[PAUSE]

Let yourself breathe in a relaxed and easy way.

[PAUSE]

In and out, let your breathing become more relaxed.

[PAUSE]

Let yourself breathe in a natural and easy way.

[PAUSE]

As you inhale, gently arch and stretch your back, extending your stomach and chest out slightly.

[PAUSE]

Let your head tilt back slightly.

[PAUSE]

(continued)

TABLE 3.10 *(continued)*

Let your lungs fill completely with refreshing and renewing air.

[PAUSE]

When you are ready, exhale and relax.

[PAUSE]

Return to a comfortable upright position.

[PAUSE]

Gently tilt your head forward.

[PAUSE]

Once again, very easily breathe in.

As you inhale, gently lean back, extending your stomach and chest out slightly.

[PAUSE]

Let your head tilt back slightly

[PAUSE]

Let your lungs fill completely with refreshing and renewing air.

[PAUSE]

When you are ready, smoothly and gently exhale and relax.

[PAUSE]

Slowly return to a comfortable upright position.

[PAUSE]

And continue breathing this way for a while.

[PAUSE 10 SECONDS]

Bowing and Breathing

Now, let your arms hang by your sides.

[PAUSE]

TABLE 3.10   *(continued)*

Make sure you are seated in an upright position.

[PAUSE]

Let your arms hang limply.

[PAUSE]

Take in a deep refreshing breath.

[PAUSE]

When you are ready to exhale, gently and slowly bow over in your chair, letting your chest and head move toward your knees.

[PAUSE]

Let gravity pull you down, slowly and easily squeezing all the air out.

[PAUSE]

When you need to take another breath, pause right where you are, gently breathe in and continue bowing and breathing out, very smoothly and gently.

[PAUSE]

And when you are ready, begin to sit up, slowly and gently.

[PAUSE]

And very easily breathe in.

[PAUSE]

Bowing, Stretching, and Breathing

This time, as you inhale, slowly and smoothly reach and stretch your arms into the air in front of you. As you breathe in, reach higher and higher to the sky.

[PAUSE]

Do this very slowly and gracefully.

[PAUSE]

(continued)

TABLE 3.10   *(continued)*

If you need to exhale, that's okay. Briefly pause where you are and smoothly let the air out. Then continue.

[PAUSE]

As you inhale, resume stretching.

[PAUSE]

Continue breathing this way until your stretch is complete.

[PAUSE]

When you are ready to unstretch and exhale, slowly circle your arms down as you breathe out.

[PAUSE]

Gently bow forward in your chair, while breathing out.

[PAUSE]

Let gravity pull your body down. There is nothing you have to do. Let your arms hang.

[PAUSE]

If you need to breathe in, that's OK. Gently pause, take in a breath of air, very smoothly and gently, and resume bowing.

[PAUSE]

Until you are bowing all the way.

[PAUSE]

Continue breathing this way, breathing in while stretching and reaching up and breathing out while bowing over. You may pause from time to time for a breath.

[PAUSE]

ACTIVE DIAPHRAGMATIC BREATHING

Stomach Squeeze Diaphragmatic Breathing

Sit up in your chair and open your hands and fingers and place them over your stomach.

[PAUSE]

TABLE 3.10 *(continued)*

Spread your fingers comfortably apart so that they cover your entire stomach, with your thumbs touch the bottom part of your chest.

[PAUSE]

Now, very easily, take a full breath, filling your stomach and chest completely. And when you are ready to exhale, firmly press in with your hands and fingers, squeezing in as if you were squeezing the air out of your abdomen.

[PAUSE]

And when you are ready to inhale, gradually release your fingers and let your stomach relax and breathe in as if your stomach were filling with air.

[PAUSE]

Breathe easily and completely.

[PAUSE]

Now continue breathing this way, squeezing your stomach as you are breathing out and relaxing your fingers as you breathe in.

[PAUSE]

Take your time.

[PAUSE]

Breathe very gently and very easily.

[PAUSE]

Focus on what it feels like to breathe completely and fully. Notice the awareness that breathing brings.

[PAUSE]

At your own pace, continue breathing evenly in and evenly out. Do not hurry. Take your time.

[PAUSE]

Focus on the even flow of air as it rushes in and out of your lungs.

[PAUSE]

Now, when you are ready, exhale and relax your fingers.

(continued)

TABLE 3.10   *(continued)*

Stomach Touch Diaphragmatic Breathing

Sit up in your chair and open your hands and fingers, again placing them over your stomach.

[PAUSE]

Spread your fingers comfortably apart so that they cover your entire stomach, with your thumbs touching the bottom part of your chest.

[PAUSE]

Let your hands and fingers remain relaxed.

[PAUSE]

As you breathe in, let the air come in on its own, as if it were filling your stomach.

[PAUSE]

Feel the stomach filling, like a large, soft balloon, filling completely.

[PAUSE]

And when you are ready to exhale, keep your fingers and hands relaxed. Let the air flow out on its own, gently and slowly.

[PAUSE]

Continue breathing this way.

[PAUSE 10 SECONDS]

Book Breathing (*Optional. Omit when taping.*)

Begin by taking and opening a hardback book.

[PAUSE]

Open it up so you can see the pages, as if you were going to read it.

[PAUSE]

Now, place the open book over your stomach so that the pages touch your stomach and the back of the book points away from your stomach.

TABLE 3.10 *(continued)*

[PAUSE]

Make sure the book is securely balanced on your stomach.

[PAUSE]

And relax.

[PAUSE]

Let your breathing be slow and easy.

[PAUSE]

Take your time.

[PAUSE]

While looking at your book, take in a slow, easy breath.

[PAUSE]

See if you can breathe in so that the book rises up.

[PAUSE]

See if you can breathe out so that the book gently falls.

[PAUSE]

Take your time.

[PAUSE]

Breathe slowly and easily.

[PAUSE]

Breathe in, book rises; breathe out, book sinks.

[PAUSE]

Continue breathing this way.

[PAUSE 10 SECONDS]

(continued)

TABLE 3.10   *(continued)*

PASSIVE BREATHING

Inhaling Through Nose

And now, rest your hands comfortably in your lap.

[PAUSE]

Let yourself relax.

[PAUSE]

Continue breathing easily and gently.

[PAUSE]

Let the flow of breath be smooth and even.

[PAUSE]

As you breathe in, imagine you are sniffing a very delicate flower.

[PAUSE]

Let the flow of breath into your nose be as smooth and gentle as possible so that you barely rustle a petal.

[PAUSE]

Take a full breath.

[PAUSE]

And relax, letting yourself breathe out slowly and naturally, without effort.

[PAUSE]

Continue breathing this way, breathing in and out quietly and evenly at your own pace.

[PAUSE]

Calmly focus on the clear inner calm that comes when you breathe in a way that is slow, full, and even.

TABLE 3.10 *(continued)*

[PAUSE]

Notice the refreshing and energizing rush of air as it quietly moves in and out of your lungs.

[PAUSE]

See how far you can follow the inward flow of air.

[PAUSE]

Can you feel it move past your nostrils?

[PAUSE]

Can you feel the air in the passages of your nose?

[PAUSE]

Can you feel the renewing and refreshing air flow into your body?

[PAUSE]

Take your time.

[PAUSE]

Breathe easily and fully.

[PAUSE]

Let yourself be fully aware of your breathing.

[PAUSE]

Continue breathing this way.

[PAUSE 10 SECONDS]

Exhaling Through Lips

Take a slow, deep breath and pause.

[PAUSE]

And breathe out slowly though your lips, as if you were blowing at a candle flame just enough to make it flicker but not go out.

(continued)

TABLE 3.10   *(continued)*

Continue breathing out, emptying all the air from your stomach and chest.

[PAUSE]

Then breathe in through your nose.

[PAUSE]

Continue breathing this way, making the stream of air that passes through your lips as you exhale as smooth and gentle as possible.

[PAUSE]

Let tension flow out with every breath.

[PAUSE]

Let the gentle movement of air dissolve any feelings of tension you might have.

[PAUSE]

Focus on the easy flow of air in as it refreshes and renews.

[PAUSE]

Let each breath fill you with peace and calm energy.

[PAUSE]

Let yourself breathe fully and evenly.

[PAUSE]

Continue breathing this way.

[PAUSE 10 SECONDS]

Occasional Deep Breaths

Let yourself breathe easily and naturally.

[PAUSE]

When you are ready, take in a full deep breath, filling your lungs and abdomen with good, refreshing air.

TABLE 3.10 *(continued)*

[PAUSE]

And when you are ready, relax.

[PAUSE]

And slowly let the air flow out, very smoothly and gently.

[PAUSE]

And now, just continue breathing normally for a while.

[PAUSE]

Do not attempt to force yourself to breathe in any particular way.

[PAUSE]

Just let the air come in and out on its own.

[PAUSE 10 SECONDS]

And, again, when you are ready, take in a full deep breath, filling your lungs with good, energizing air. Feel the calm and strength it brings.

[PAUSE]

And, when ready, gently and smoothly exhale.

[PAUSE]

Then resume breathing in a normal way, easily in and out.

[PAUSE 10 SECONDS]

Focused Breathing

Breath in a relaxed manner, in and out through your nose.

[PAUSE]

Try not to force your breathing.

[PAUSE]

Become fully aware of the air as it rushes in and out, flowing into and out of your lungs.

(continued)

TABLE 3.10 *(continued)*

[PAUSE]

Filling your body with refreshing and renewing air.

[PAUSE]

Calmly focus on the unhurried rhythm of your breathing. Let yourself breathe effortlessly, without strain.

[PAUSE 10 SECONDS]

Focus on the even flow of air as it moves in and out of your lungs through your nose.

[PAUSE 10 SECONDS]

Notice how the easy flow of energizes and relaxes you.

[PAUSE]

The flow of air brings peace and inner strength.

[PAUSE]

Continue breathing this way for a while.

[PAUSE 10 SECONDS]

And gently let go of what you are attending to.

[PAUSE]

Slowly open your eyes.

[PAUSE]

We have completed our breathing exercise.

APPROACH 4: YOGAFORM STRETCHING

Yoga stretching is a popular approach to relaxation with ancient roots. Traditional yoga exercises number in the thousands and have deep ties to religion and philosophy. We focus on hatha yoga, an approach that emphasizes simple stretching. Although hatha yoga is derived from a rich philosophical tradition, the exercises we present are simple stretches; for this reason we call our approach yogaform stretching. Spiritual, religious, and metaphysical references have been avoided. Potentially dangerous and superfluous exercises have not been included. Generally, our approach incorporates only the exercises that are mentioned most frequently in introductory yoga texts and have a record of ease and enjoyability.

In my experience, yogaform stretching appears to enhance R-States of Mental Relaxation and Strength and Awareness and should be used when greater alertness and awareness is desired (Smith et al., 1996). Stretching exercises may be fairly effective for reducing high levels of skeletal muscle tension to an "average" baseline. They are perhaps less effective for sustained and deep reductions in physiological arousal below baseline, given that beginning hatha exercises require sustained skeletal arousal to maintain a posture or stretch. If my speculations are correct, autogenic suggestions and simple yogaform stretching would be an inappropriate match.

Although a moderate amount of research has considered the impact of yoga, much is of questionable value (Funderburk, 1977). The most cited studies (Patel, 1993; Vahia, Doongaji, Jeste, Ravindranath, Kapoor, & Ardhapurkar, 1973) have combined stretching, breathing, imagery, meditation, philosophical discussion, and even PMR, a technique that tends to evoke quite different R-States. Thus, it is difficult to assess the source of any effects obtained. In addition, many studies have considered hatha yoga as a physical fitness or rehabilitation exercise, measuring flexibility, respiratory capacity and efficiency, circulation, and the like. The impact of yoga stretching on such variables is, of course, beyond the consideration of this book. Finally, occasional lifelong practitioners of yoga stretching have demonstrated dramatic abilities to lower heart rate and breathing rate. Impressive as such feats of self-control may appear, their generalizability to most practitioners and their implications for relaxation are unclear.

Easy yogaform stretches are easier to teach than PMR, with less likelihood of mishap or incorrect practice. Thus, although the clinical effect of yogaform stretching is still subject to research, the exercises may be applied on a trial-and-error basis with relative safety. Patel (1993) recommends not applying yoga-based therapy "in most cases of malignant or secondary hypertension, in view of the critical nature of these conditions. It should also not be used in depressive or psychotic patients" (p. 111). I disagree in part and suggest that mild stretches can be applied with careful clinical supervision. One can make a case that exercises that evoke Strength and Awareness might be well suited for depressed clients. This is an important empirical question.

When presenting yogaform stretching, moderate your voice to suggest the act of slowly stretching and unstretching. Elongate vowels ("Sloooowly stretch"). Speak as if you were stretching yourself. Avoid at all costs a PMR or AT monotone. The yoga voice should be relaxed, calm, and refreshed, suggesting calm alertness.

Step 1: Explanation and Rationale

It is perhaps appropriate to avoid the excessive claims often found in popular yoga manuals ("yoga will . . . stimulate your liver, cleanse your blood, heighten your senses," etc.). Instead, I recommend describing yoga stretches as one approach to reducing muscle tension. Here is one rationale I use (Smith, 1989):

> A tense muscle can be likened to a tightly coiled spring. If we wanted to loosen the spring we could easily stretch it out and then release the stretch. Similarly, in the yogaform exercises we slowly, smoothly, and gently stretch each muscle, and then easily release the stretch. (p. 84)

If a client also has been taught PMR, it is useful to differentiate how the process of stretching is different from tensing and letting go:

> The process is quite different from that involved in PMR. The most obvious difference is that PMR exercises involve rapid constriction followed by 20 to 30 seconds of inactivity, whereas the yogaform exercises involve continuous smooth movement—stretching and unstretching.
>
> However, there are other differences that are a bit more subtle. A smooth and continuous stretch requires us to focus our attention for the duration of the stretch; squeezing requires relatively less sustained attention. This point can be easily illustrated. Quickly make a fist and then let go. That action required little focused attention. Indeed, we often "clench up" automatically when threatened. Now, slowly open your fingers. Do this very slowly, smoothly, and gently, as if there were feathers resting on each

finger. Notice how you had to attend more carefully to your fingers. By focusing your attention in a sustained manner you will be developing an important relaxation skill. (Smith, 1989, p. 84)

Step 2: Demonstration

Proceed to demonstrate each yoga stretch you wish to teach. Practice in an alert seated position (feet flat on floor, spine and neck erect), or standing up. Table 3.11 presents instructions for the following exercises:

Hand stretch

Arm stretch

Arm and side stretch

Back stretch

Shoulder stretch

Back of neck stretch

Face stretch

Front of neck stretch

Stomach and chest stretch

Leg stretch

Foot stretch

Emphasize that each stretch is to be done slowly, smoothly, and gently, in contrast to PMR. For each exercise, take about 20 seconds to stretch the indicated muscle group. When a muscle is stretched, have the client hold the stretch and attend to the pleasant sensations for a few seconds. Then take about 20 seconds to unstretch. Have the client move as slowly, smoothly, and gently as possible, keeping the mind focused on the movement and the sensations produced. Do each exercise twice. For each done on the right side, repeat on the left.

Steps 3, 4, and 5: Dress Rehearsal, Checking, and Modification

Present the entire sequence as described. The stretching exercises here are relatively easy and enjoyable, and they rarely cause problems. At times clients want to speed up (or perhaps slow down) the pace of presentation. Try to maintain as slow a pace as the client can tolerate. Emphasize that the point is to create a pleasurable stretch, not an athletic or heroic stretch or a stretch that is painful. Clients vary considerably in how far they can stretch. Emphasize that the value of a stretch is not how far one can move but the degree to which one creates a smooth movement and a pleasurable "stretch sensation." Thus, a small stretch and a large stretch can be equally effective. Bowing and touching the floor is in itself no better than bowing a few inches.

Some clients show concerns that their movements are jerky, not completely smooth. Reassure clients that such "rusty movement" is a natural sign of being a beginner. Movement generally smooths out with practice. Go gently with the neck stretches; they can create discomfort. And finally, there is the matter of the face stretch, or as it is called in India, the "lion." In group practice, clients invariably break out in laughter when they all fully open their jaws (with extended tongue), mouths, and eyes, in public. Some yoga instructors treat such mirthfulness with solemn admonitions to "practice seriously." This is regrettable. A little humor is very good; it can contribute to an attitude of letting go in relaxation and to the R-States Mental Relaxation, Strength and Awareness, and Joy. After the laugh, try the exercise again, this time with everyone looking toward the sky.

If the full sequence of PMR exercises has already been taught, the very same muscle groups are presented in yogaform stretching. This gives the client the opportunity to compare and contrast the effects of these very different approaches.

The following are suggestions for enhancing yogaform stretching:

- Freely incorporate breathing exercises.
- Introduce imagery suggestive of the R-State Strength and Awareness, consistent with the attempted stretch. For example, when stretching one's arms to the sky, an accompanying image such as "Imagine you are a tree, with branches reaching high into the sky" would be appropriate.
- Avoid PMR and AT, given that these approaches foster R-States different from those associated with yogaform stretching.
- End with imagery or meditation.
- Practice in a setting suggestive of Strength and Awareness (e.g., a well-lit room, outdoors).

TABLE 3.11   Script for Yogaform Stretching

(Words that are in **boldface** or [BRACKETED] are special instructions to trainers. These words are not to be read or spoken to clients.)

Right Hand Stretch

We'll begin with the right hand.

Slowly, smoothly, and gently open your fingers and easily stretch them back and apart.

[PAUSE]

Try not to stretch so that it hurts.

[PAUSE]

Focus on the good feelings of stretching.

[PAUSE]

Take your time.

[PAUSE]

Stretch every muscle fully.

[PAUSE]

Then hold the stretch

[PAUSE]

And slowly, smoothly, and gently release the stretch.

[PAUSE]

Let your fingers very slowly return to their original relaxed position.

[PAUSE]

Notice the sensations as the muscles unstretch.

[PAUSE]

Take your time; there is no need to hurry.

(continued)

TABLE 3.11 *(continued)*

[PAUSE]

Right Hand Stretch (Repeat)

Now let's try that again.

[PAUSE]

Without hurrying, very easily and gently open the fingers of your right hand.

[PAUSE]

Open them wide apart so that you can feel a full and comfortable stretch.

[PAUSE]

Let each finger open more and more.

[PAUSE]

Let yourself become aware of the sensations of stretching.

[PAUSE]

Then hold the stretch.

[PAUSE]

Then slowly, smoothly, and gently release the stretch.

[PAUSE]

Let your movement be smooth.

[PAUSE]

Take your time.

[PAUSE]

Easily return your fingers to their original position.

[PAUSE]

TABLE 3.11   *(continued)*

Left Hand Stretch

We're now ready to move to the other hand.

[PAUSE]

Slowly, smoothly, and gently open the fingers.

[PAUSE]

Move them farther and farther apart.

[PAUSE]

Make sure your right hand remains relaxed.

[PAUSE]

Open them more and more so that you feel a good compete stretch.

[PAUSE]

Then hold the stretch.

[PAUSE]

And gently and easily release your fingers.

[PAUSE]

Let your fingers gently and smoothly return to their resting position.

[PAUSE]

There is no need to hurry.

[PAUSE]

Move at a pace that feels comfortable for you.

[PAUSE]

Left Hand Stretch (Repeat)

And let's try that once again.

(continued)

TABLE 3.11   *(continued)*

[PAUSE]

Very easily and gently open the fingers.

[PAUSE]

Notice how it feels as your fingers stretch farther apart.

[PAUSE]

Let the movement be smooth and graceful.

[PAUSE]

Each finger farther and farther apart.

[PAUSE]

And hold the stretch.

[PAUSE]

Do not hurry or rush.

[PAUSE]

Let your arm relax and return.

[PAUSE]

Notice the pleasant sensations of stretching and relaxing.

[PAUSE]

And gently and easily release the stretch.

[PAUSE]

Let the fingers gently return.

[PAUSE]

Try not to hurry or rush.

[PAUSE]

Notice the peaceful and refreshing feelings of relaxation.

[PAUSE]

Right Arm Stretch

Rest your right hand comfortably on your right leg.

[PAUSE]

TABLE 3.11 *(continued)*

Now move to your right arm.

[PAUSE]

Slowly, smoothly, and gently slide your hand down your leg.

[PAUSE]

Extend your arm farther and farther, slowly stretching out in front of you.

[PAUSE]

Reach out and extend your arm in front of you.

[PAUSE]

Very gracefully, as if you are balancing a feather on each hand.

[PAUSE]

And hold the stretch and become aware of the sensations.

[PAUSE]

Then slowly, smoothly, and gently return your hand.

[PAUSE]

Slide your hand back.

[PAUSE]

Gently rest your hand on your leg and slide your arm back to its resting position.

[PAUSE]

Take your time.

[PAUSE]

Slowly and gently unstretch your arm.

[PAUSE]

Right Arm Stretch (Repeat)

And once again, slowly, smoothly, and gently slide your hand down your leg.

(continued)

TABLE 3.11 *(continued)*

[PAUSE]

Reach and stretch. Open your arm more and more.

[PAUSE]

Reach out in front of you.

[PAUSE]

Feel a full and comfortable stretch.

[PAUSE]

And hold the stretch.

[PAUSE]

Then gently an easily return your arm.

[PAUSE]

Left Arm Stretch

Now move to your other arm.

[PAUSE]

Once again, quietly and easily reach and stretch.

[PAUSE]

Let your hand slide down your leg.

[PAUSE]

Stretch more and more so that you are fully aware of a full and comfortable stretch.

[PAUSE]

Make sure your right arm remains relaxed.

[PAUSE]

Then hold the stretch.

[PAUSE]

TABLE 3.11 *(continued)*

And slowly and easily let your arm return.

[PAUSE]

Take your time.

[PAUSE]

Let the hand and arm gently and gracefully unstretch.

[PAUSE]

Notice the sensations of stretching and unstretching.

[PAUSE]

Left Arm Stretch (Repeat)

Now, once again, reach and stretch.

[PAUSE]

Slowly, smoothly, and gently.

[PAUSE]

Make a full and comfortable stretch.

[PAUSE]

Focus on the sensations of stretching.

[PAUSE]

And hold the stretch.

[PAUSE]

Then easily return your arm.

[PAUSE]

Let it slide back to its resting position.

[PAUSE]

Very smoothly and easily.

(continued)

TABLE 3.11 *(continued)*

[PAUSE]

Let it relax.

[PAUSE]

Right Arm and Side Stretch

Now let both your arms fall limply to your sides.

[PAUSE]

Slowly, smoothly, and gently circle your right arm and hand up and away from your body like the hand of a clock or the wing of a bird.

[PAUSE]

Let your arm extend straight, and circle higher and higher.

[PAUSE]

Let it circle to the sky.

[PAUSE]

And then circle your arm over your head so that your hand points to the other side . . . and arch your body as you reach and point farther and farther, like a tree arching in the wind.

[PAUSE]

Become aware of the invigorating feelings of stretching.

[PAUSE]

Now gently and easily,

[PAUSE]

Like the hand of a clock or the wing of a bird

[PAUSE]

Circle your arm back over your head . . . to your side

[PAUSE]

Finally to the resting position.

TABLE 3.11 *(continued)*

[PAUSE]

And let your arm hang.

[PAUSE]

Right Arm and Side Stretch (Repeat)

Let's do that once again.

[PAUSE]

Circle your arm.

[PAUSE]

Very easily and gently, up to the side.

[PAUSE]

Higher and higher, over your head.

[PAUSE]

Pointing to the other side.

[PAUSE]

Reaching and stretching farther and farther.

[PAUSE]

Feel a full and comfortable stretch in your entire body as it arches.

[PAUSE]

Then slowly circle your arm back.

[PAUSE]

Evenly and gently without rushing.

[PAUSE]

Like the hand of a clock or the wing of a bird.

(continued)

TABLE 3.11 *(continued)*

[PAUSE]

Take your time.

[PAUSE]

Easily return your arm to your side and let it hang again.

[PAUSE]

Left Arm and Side Stretch

Now the other side.

[PAUSE]

Smoothly and gently circle your arm and hand up to your side.

[PAUSE]

Like the hand of a clock or the wing of a bird.

[PAUSE]

Let it reach higher and higher.

[PAUSE]

Until it is pointing to the sky.

[PAUSE]

And reach and stretch to the other side.

[PAUSE]

Become aware of the refreshing feelings of stretching all along your body.

[PAUSE]

Hold the stretch.

[PAUSE]

Then slowly and easily,

TABLE 3.11 *(continued)*

[PAUSE]

Like the hand of a clock or the wing of a bird,

[PAUSE]

Circle your arm back to the side.

[PAUSE]

Gracefully and gently let it circle down.

[PAUSE]

Try not to hurry.

[PAUSE]

And return your arm to your side.

[PAUSE]

Let yourself relax and your mind become peacefully clear.

[PAUSE]

Left Arm and Side Stretch (Repeat)

Once again.

[PAUSE]

Very easily and gently,

[PAUSE]

Circle your arm up, higher and higher,

[PAUSE]

Up to your side,

[PAUSE]

Gradually over your head, pointing up.

[PAUSE]

(continued)

TABLE 3.11 *(continued)*

Reach to the other side, and feel a full and comfortable stretch.

[PAUSE]

Then gently release the stretch.

[PAUSE]

Gently return your arm.

[PAUSE]

Like the hand of a clock or the wing of a bird.

[PAUSE]

Slowly and gently to the side.

[PAUSE]

Lower and lower.

[PAUSE]

Until your arm is again hanging comfortably by your side.

[PAUSE]

And enjoy the feelings of energy and calm you have released.

[HALFWAY POINT]

Back Stretch

Now focus your attention on your back, below your shoulders.

[PAUSE]

Slowly, smoothly, and gently relax and bow over.

[PAUSE]

Let your arms hang limply.

[PAUSE]

Let your head fall forward, as you bow forward farther and farther in your chair.

TABLE 3.11 *(continued)*

[PAUSE]

Do not force yourself to bow over. . . . Let gravity pull your body toward your knees . . . farther and farther. It's OK to take a short breath if you need to.

[PAUSE]

Feel the stretch along the back.

[PAUSE]

Let gravity pull your body forward, as far as it will go.

[PAUSE]

Then gently and easily sit up.

[PAUSE]

Take your time.

[PAUSE]

Inch by inch, straighten up your body.

[PAUSE]

Until you are seated comfortably in an upright position.

[PAUSE]

Back Stretch (Repeat)

Now again.

[PAUSE]

Let gravity pull your body down toward your knees.

[PAUSE]

Farther and farther.

[PAUSE]

Feel the stretch along your back.

[PAUSE]

(continued)

TABLE 3.11   *(continued)*

Let your entire torso bend forward, farther and farther.

[PAUSE]

Let your head hang limply.

[PAUSE]

Now gradually sit up.

[PAUSE]

Move at a pace that feels comfortable.

[PAUSE]

Gently straighten your back.

[PAUSE]

Return to your original erect position.

[PAUSE]

And make sure you are seated comfortably.

[PAUSE]

Shoulder Stretch

Now lift both arms straight ahead in front of you and let your fingers touch.

[PAUSE]

Slowly, smoothly, and gently circle them around together, as if you were squeezing a big pillow.

[PAUSE]

Slowly, let your hands cross, pointing in opposite directions.

[PAUSE]

Squeeze farther and farther so that you can feel a stretch in your shoulders and back.

[PAUSE]

TABLE 3.11 *(continued)*

Hold the stretch.

[PAUSE]

Become aware of the good sensations of stretching.

[PAUSE]

And gently release the stretch.

[PAUSE]

Gradually return your arms to your side.

[PAUSE]

Take your time; there is no need to hurry.

[PAUSE]

Let your arms relax.

[PAUSE]

Shoulder Stretch (Repeat)

Now again.

[PAUSE]

Lift both arms, and slowly, smoothly, and gently cross them in front of you.

[PAUSE]

Imagine you are squeezing a big pillow.

[PAUSE]

Stretch the shoulders and back.

[PAUSE]

Hold the stretch.

[PAUSE]

(continued)

TABLE 3.11 *(continued)*

Then gently release your arms.

[PAUSE]

Gradually return your arms to their original position.

[PAUSE]

Let your arms relax.

[PAUSE]

Move at a pace that feels comfortable.

[PAUSE]

And when you are done, rest your hands comfortably in your lap.

[PAUSE]

Back of Neck Stretch

Now, while sitting erect, let your head tilt easily toward your chest.

[PAUSE]

Try not to force it down.

[PAUSE]

Simply let gravity pull your head down.

[PAUSE]

Farther and farther.

[PAUSE]

Focus on the stretch in the back of your neck.

[PAUSE]

The refreshing and renewing energy it releases.

[PAUSE]

TABLE 3.11 *(continued)*

As the force of gravity easily and slowly pulls your head down.

[PAUSE]

When you are ready

[PAUSE]

Gently and easily lift your head.

[PAUSE]

Lift it until it is again comfortably upright.

[PAUSE]

Back of Neck Stretch (Repeat)

Now again, let gravity pull your head down.

[PAUSE]

Let your head fall farther and farther toward your chest.

[PAUSE]

Feel the muscles in the back of your neck stretch.

[PAUSE]

Do not force your head down, let your neck relax.

[PAUSE]

And let gravity do the work for you.

[PAUSE]

And when you are ready,

[PAUSE]

Gently and easily lift your head.

[PAUSE]

Gradually move your head to an upright position.

[PAUSE]

Until your head is comfortably erect.

(continued)

TABLE 3.11 *(continued)*

[PAUSE]

And enjoy the feelings of strength and calm awareness you have released.

[PAUSE]

Face Stretch

Now attend to the muscles of your face.

[PAUSE]

Slowly, smoothly, and gently open your jaws, mouth, and eyes while lifting your eyebrows.

[PAUSE]

Open wide.

[PAUSE]

Feel every muscle of your face stretch more and more.

[PAUSE]

Hold the stretch.

[PAUSE]

Then gently and easily release the stretch.

[PAUSE]

Let the muscles smooth out as they relax.

[PAUSE]

Let your face settle into a comfortable position.

[PAUSE]

Face Stretch (Repeat)

Once again, gently and easily open your jaws, mouth, and eyes.

TABLE 3.11 *(continued)*

[PAUSE]

Open them more and more so that you can feel a full and comfortable stretch in your entire face.

[PAUSE]

When you are stretching as far as you can, gently hold the stretch.

[PAUSE]

Attend to the sensations of stretching.

[PAUSE]

Then gently and easily release the stretch.

[PAUSE]

Let the muscles of the face smooth out.

[PAUSE]

Let your face muscles relax more and more.

[PAUSE]

Until they are in a relaxed and comfortable position.

[PAUSE]

Front of Neck Stretch

Now, as before, let your head tilt, this time backward.

[PAUSE]

Let gravity pull your head back, but not too far, just enough to feel the stretch.

[PAUSE]

Do not force it back.

(continued)

TABLE 3.11   *(continued)*

[PAUSE]

Let gravity do the work for you as it pulls the heavy weight of your head back farther and farther.

[PAUSE]

Gently and slightly open your mouth, and let your head relax and fall back.

[PAUSE]

Focus your mind on the front of the neck stretch as it stretches.

[PAUSE]

Gently hold the stretch.

[PAUSE]

Then gently and easily lift your head.

[PAUSE]

Gradually return it to its upright position

[PAUSE]

Take your time. There is no need to hurry.

[PAUSE]

Front of Neck Stretch (Repeat)

Now again.

[PAUSE]

Let gravity pull your head back.

[PAUSE]

Just enough to feel the stretch.

[PAUSE]

Easily and gently, so that you can feel the stretch in your neck.

TABLE 3.11 *(continued)*

[PAUSE]

Try not to exert any effort.

[PAUSE]

Just let go, and let your head gently tilt back.

[PAUSE]

Then easily and gently,

[PAUSE]

Let your head return to an upright position.

[PAUSE]

And let your head rest comfortably.

[PAUSE]

Stomach and Chest Stretch

Now lean back comfortably in your chair.

[PAUSE]

Slowly, smoothly, and gently arch your stomach and chest out.

[PAUSE]

Do this slowly and gently.

[PAUSE]

Feel a stretch along your torso.

[PAUSE]

Arch and stretch.

[PAUSE]

Then gently and easily release the stretch.

(continued)

TABLE 3.11 *(continued)*

[PAUSE]

Slowly and easily return to an upright position.

[PAUSE]

Take your time. There is no reason to hurry.

[PAUSE]

Stomach and Chest Stretch (Repeat)

And again.

[PAUSE]

Slowly and easily arch your stomach and chest out.

[PAUSE]

Arch your back more and more.

[PAUSE]

Feel a full and comfortable stretch all along your torso.

[PAUSE]

Then gently and easily release the stretch.

[PAUSE]

Gradually return your back to its original position.

[PAUSE]

And sit comfortably in an upright position.

[PAUSE]

Right Leg Stretch

Now focus your attention on your right leg.

[PAUSE]

TABLE 3.11 *(continued)*

Slowly and easily stretch the leg out in front of you.

[PAUSE]

Stretch and twist so that you can feel the muscles pulling.

[PAUSE]

Do this easily and gently.

[PAUSE]

Feel a good energizing stretch all along your leg.

[PAUSE]

Then gently release the stretch.

[PAUSE]

Slowly let your leg return to its original resting position.

[PAUSE]

Take your time.

[PAUSE]

Gently unstretch your leg.

[PAUSE]

And let it rest.

[PAUSE]

Right Leg Stretch (Repeat)

Now once again, easily and gently stretch your leg out.

[PAUSE]

Easily and gently, stretch farther and farther.

[PAUSE]

(continued)

TABLE 3.11   *(continued)*

Notice the stimulating sensation of stretching.

[PAUSE]

Then hold the stretch.

[PAUSE]

Now slowly and easily unstretch.

[PAUSE]

Let the leg easily return.

[PAUSE]

Take your time. There is no need to hurry.

[PAUSE]

Notice the sensations of unstretching.

[PAUSE]

Left Leg Stretch

Now focus on your left leg.

[PAUSE]

Slowly and evenly stretch the leg out.

[PAUSE]

Feel every muscle pulling and stretching.

[PAUSE]

Notice the pleasant sensations associated with stretching.

[PAUSE]

Stretch all the way.

[PAUSE]

And hold the stretch.

TABLE 3.11   *(continued)*

[PAUSE]

Now easily and gently release the stretch.

[PAUSE]

Take your time.

[PAUSE]

Release the stretch very gently.

[PAUSE]

Return your leg to its original resting position.

[PAUSE]

Left Leg Stretch (Repeat)

Now, once again, gently and easily stretch.

[PAUSE]

Stretch the leg out farther and farther.

[PAUSE]

Feel the sensations of stretching.

[PAUSE]

Take your time stretching.

[PAUSE]

And hold the stretch.

[PAUSE]

Now gently release the stretch.

(continued)

TABLE 3.11 *(continued)*

[PAUSE]

Inch by inch, move your leg back to its resting position.

[PAUSE]

Move your leg as smoothly as possible.

[PAUSE]

Notice the sensations associated with unstretching.

[PAUSE]

Right Foot Stretch

Now focus your attention on your right foot.

[PAUSE]

While resting your heel on the floor, gently pull your toes and foot up, as if they were being pulled by strings

[PAUSE]

Let the foot and leg stretch more and more.

[PAUSE]

Feel the full and comfortable stretch in every muscle fiber.

[PAUSE]

Stretch all the way.

[PAUSE]

And hold the stretch.

[PAUSE]

Now, easily and gently, release the stretch.

[PAUSE]

Let the foot slowly and smoothly relax.

[PAUSE]

TABLE 3.11 *(continued)*

Inch by inch, let the foot return.

[PAUSE]

Unstretch the foot until it is resting again on the floor.

[PAUSE]

Right Foot Stretch (Repeat)

Once again, slowly lift the foot and toes, resting your heel on the floor.

[PAUSE]

Feel the stretch all along your foot and leg.

[PAUSE]

Feel a full and comfortable stretch.

[PAUSE]

Slowly and gently.

[PAUSE]

And hold the stretch.

[PAUSE]

Now gently lower the foot.

[PAUSE]

Easily return the foot.

[PAUSE]

Take your time, return your foot gently.

[PAUSE]

And let your foot relax.

[PAUSE]

(continued)

TABLE 3.11 *(continued)*

Left Foot Stretch

Now focus your attention on your left foot.

[PAUSE]

Imagine strings are pulling your left toes and foot up.

[PAUSE]

Stretch the foot, toes, and leg, more and more.

[PAUSE]

Feel the stretch all along your foot and leg.

[PAUSE]

Feel a full and comfortable stretch.

[PAUSE]

And hold the stretch.

[PAUSE]

Then slowly release the stretch.

[PAUSE]

Gently relax the toes and foot.

[PAUSE]

Slowly lower them to the floor.

[PAUSE]

Take your time. Go easily and gently.

[PAUSE]

Left Foot Stretch (Repeat)

Once again, stretch the left foot and toes up.

TABLE 3.11   *(continued)*

[PAUSE]

Stretch more and more.

[PAUSE]

Feel every muscle stretching.

[PAUSE]

Notice the sensations of stretching.

[PAUSE]

And hold the sketch.

[PAUSE]

Then slowly and gently release the stretch.

[PAUSE]

Without hurrying, lower the foot.

[PAUSE]

Inch by inch, let the foot return to the floor.

[PAUSE]

And let the foot and leg relax in a resting position.

[PAUSE]

And let go of what you are attending to.

[PAUSE]

Slowly open your eyes, if they are closed.

[PAUSE]

We have completed our relaxation exercise.

APPROACH 5: IMAGERY

I find it useful to define imagery as the covert (or mental) generation of any activity or setting one finds relaxing. The one exception is autogenic preparatory imagery, which has a client attend to the visual effects of spontaneous retinal phenomena (phosphene activity) that are often apparent with eyes closed. I suggest three general categories of imagery: sense, narrative, and insight. In sense imagery, one simply imagines sensations associated with a relaxing activity or setting. I suggest involving all senses, rather than simply vision. The four categories of stimuli I have found most useful include travel imagery (boats, plains, trains, balloons, horses), outdoor setting imagery (mountains, gardens, forests), water imagery (rivers, lakes, ocean beach, rain), and indoor imagery (childhood home, castle, religious institution, cabin). Of these, water imagery tends to be most preferred. In contrast to sense imagery, narrative imagery emphasizes a relaxing activity rather than sensations. It is a type of imagery that depicts a simple relaxing activity story, without an ending.

Finally, insight imagery has a story or plot with a singular, engaging concluding focus. After a brief narration (walking through the woods, climbing a mountain, entering a deep cave, etc.), the relaxer encounters a simple stimulus (pond, rock, closed magic box, etc.). He or she is told to passively and nonanalytically contemplate this stimulus, to quietly focus and let associative thoughts or images arise, sometimes as related to a specific question or issue. For example, one might be told: "Attend to the secret box. This box contains a response to your question. Wait for it to open and present you with its response."

I have developed a variation of insight imagery that incorporates a client's R-Beliefs, or personal philosophies conducive to deepened and generalized relaxation. In *R-Belief Imagery* a client is first presented with the Smith R-Beliefs Inventory (SRBI, in Appendix). This scale simply lists affirmations that research has found to be most associated with relaxation. Clients are instructed simply to browse through the list, rather than evaluate each item as if it were an exam. Initial presentation of the SRBI serves to "prime the pump," or establish subtle expectancies for the ensuing exercise. The client is then guided through preparatory sense imagery (relaxing travel) to a relaxing place (outdoor pond with a wise person in the distance). Here, formal imagery begins. The client simply entertains an image of this setting, recognizing the possibility that a "message of calm and peace" may appear in any of a number of ways. The message may appear reflected on the pond. The wise person in the distance may approach and speak the message. Or perhaps the peaceful setting in and of itself reflects a message of calm and peace. It is important not to create a demand that the message "must appear." Initial exposure to the SRBI is usually sufficient to enable clients to recognize the manifestation of their relaxation beliefs in a beautiful and peaceful setting.

Imagery also varies according to degree of trainer guidance and structure. Some clients prefer guided and structured imagery in which a trainer continues to present details of an imagery script. Such imagery is not unlike simple storytelling. In contrast, with unguided and unstructured imagery, a trainer presents the bare beginnings of an imagery theme and lets the client proceed with imagery in silence. I prefer an intermediate level of trainer guidance and structure in which a variety of imagery script options are outlined and the client is given considerable leeway to elaborate. Complete scripts for sense and insight imagery are presented in Tables 3.12 and 3.13.

Imagery exercises are similar to fantasy and should be accessible to a wide range of clients. I suspect imagery tends to evoke the R-States Joy, Love and Thankfulness, Prayerfulness, and perhaps Disengagement. Insight imagery requires a degree of focusing ability and is perhaps less appropriate for clients who are easily distracted or need a highly structured and familiar training format. Currently, there is little evidence as to the superiority of imagery over other approaches.

The voice quality appropriate for imagery depends on whether it fosters withdrawal or opening up. Disengaging talk should be quiet and rather monotonous. Talk designed to enhance R-States related to opening up should be a bit more "colorful," with inflections corresponding to key story phrases. Such engaging talk is not unlike the storytelling voice one might employ in telling an interesting story to a child.

Step 1: Explanation and Rationale

It is important to differentiate between types of imagery and to point out that relaxation imagery is different from the problem-focused imagery and mental rehearsal one might deploy in preparation for a stressful situation. In relaxation imagery one mentally creates or re-creates an activity or setting that one feels is relaxing. Explain that the first steps are to select a topic and then fill in the sense details.

Steps 2 and 3: Demonstration, Dress Rehearsal

This book offers scripted instructions for sense imagery and insight imagery. The sense imagery script invites a client to enjoy a pleasant "fantasy daydream." Brief sample images are offered for four themes: travel, outdoor/nature, water, and indoor. A client then selects the theme of his or her image and suggests sense details (what is seen, heard, touched, and smelled). The instructor then presents the chosen theme, including the sense details offered by the client. For the remaining 10 minutes of silence, the client silently engages in imagery.

The insight imagery script invites the client to imagine an interesting story, one that has a relaxing message. The trainer presents three possible themes from which to choose, one involving travel, one a magic pond, and one a wise person. At the end of each theme, the client is invited to find a "special, relaxing message." The client selects a theme from the three presented, fills in the sense details (as in sense imagery), and for 10 minutes silently engages in imagery.

Steps 4 and 5: Checking, Modification

The most serious problem with most forms of imagery (especially standardized or taped imagery) is the "booby trap," an unanticipated problem association that emerges after imagery has begun. For example, a client may have chosen beach imagery, only to realize, in the middle of the imagery task, that beaches remind him of the time he was seriously sunburned. After dress rehearsal, it is important to describe the concept of the booby trap and to revise the selected image if any are thought of.

In addition, clients may complain of difficulty in producing vivid, lifelike images. Unlike programs such as AT, which encourage and value images that are vivid as possible, I reassure clients that they can enjoy an image even if visuals are not vivid or even are absent. After all, one can enjoy a good story without accompanying illustrations.

Finally, clients differ in how much "trainer talk" they prefer. It is important to ask clients if you should incorporate more or less verbal description in your imagery presentation.

The following are suggestions for enhancing imagery:

- Any form of relaxation can precede imagery instructions.
- Simple, nonintrusive variations of any exercise can be incorporated into an imagery theme. Examples:
    "Imagine you are an autumn leaf holding onto a tree. Gently tense up your hands (PMR). As a relaxing breeze flows by, let go (PMR) and float to earth."

"Imagine you are in a warm, relaxing pond of water. Notice how you feel warm and heavy (AT)."

"Imagine a relaxing cloud floating overhead. A gentle breeze moves the cloud along. Breathe in the refreshing air and exhale."

- End imagery with meditation. If you do this, gradually introduce imagery suggestions that are increasingly passive, simple, and focused. Select a meditation focal stimulus consistent with the image. (See "Deepening Imagery" in chapter 4.) Example: "Imagine a wonderful pond. You can see birds and clouds in the air, feel the cool breeze against your skin, and hear the bubbling water. As evening approaches, things grow quiet. The clouds float away. The birds become silent. The air and water are still. And all you see in front of you is the simple pond, like a round mirror reflecting the dark night sky. Meditate on this pond."
- Select an interesting and relaxing setting evocative of imagery.

TABLE 3.12   Script for Sense Imagery

(Words that are in **boldface** or [BRACKETED] are special instructions to trainers. These words are not to be read or spoken to clients.)

RATIONALE/EXPLANATION

In this exercise we are going to learn to relax with a special type of daydream or fantasy. Daydreaming and fantasy can provide a very relaxing break from the tensions of the day. However, in order for this to work best, you first need to do two things. First, select a special type of theme, one that is specially relaxing to you. Second, pick details for your fantasy theme. In today's session, I will first guide you on a fantasy journey and demonstrate four different types of themes. Next, you pick which image you liked best. We will close with a 10-minute fantasy/daydream exercise.

First, make sure you are seated upright in a comfortable position. Are your feet resting comfortably on the floor?

[PAUSE ABOUT 30 SECONDS FOR CLIENT OR GROUP TO RELAX.]

DEMONSTRATION

In our minds we will take a special fantasy journey. We will travel to a relaxing place, far away from the cares of the world, and enjoy

(continued)

TABLE 3.12   *(continued)*

what it has to offer. Travel can be very relaxing to many people. In your mind you can move far away from the cares of the day. You might want to think about floating high in the air in a balloon. Can you see the clouds float by? Far below is the world floating past. The relaxing air touches your skin. You can hear the relaxing sound of wind brushing against the balloon. You can smell the clean air around you.

Or you might imagine yourself in a boat floating far out to sea. You can see the distant trees. You can hear the gentle sound of waves lapping against your boat. The water touches your skin. The smell of the water is very peaceful. Your cares are very distant.

Or you might imagine yourself moving through a remote country-side in a train. You can see the pastures rushing past. The creaking sound of the train on the tracks has a soothing quality about it. You smell the wood in the train. You can feel the gentle swaying motion.

For the next minute or so let yourself enjoy a daydream about traveling. Let yourself become more and more distant from the cares of the day. You are in your own fantasy world. Involve all of your senses. What do you see? What do you hear? What do you feel touching your skin? What do you smell?

[PAUSE 1 MINUTE]

Gently let go of what you are attending to.

We are ready to move on.

In our relaxing journey of the mind, we have arrived at a distant land, a faraway peaceful place outdoors. You might picture your-self on the top of a mountain. You can see far into the distance. You can hear the songs of birds echoing. You can feel the crisp mountain air. And the mountain pines smell fresh and relaxing.

You might picture a faraway grassy plain. Waves of grass extend into the distance. You can hear the wind rushing through the meadow. You can feel the soft grass touching your skin. Its peace-ful and refreshing fragrance fills the air.

Or you might think of a valley. All around are towering moun-tains. You are next to a giant forest. You can hear the chirping of squirrels. You can feel the warm mountain sun. And you smell the gentle fragrance of flowers.

For the next minute or so let yourself enjoy a daydream about a faraway peaceful outdoor setting of your own. Involve all of your senses.

[PAUSE 1 MINUTE]

TABLE 3.12 *(continued)*

Gently let go of what you are attending to.

We are ready to move on.

There are many peaceful and relaxing things to enjoy in your relaxing setting. Some may involve the theme of water. What relaxing water setting can you imagine?

You might imagine yourself floating in a pond. You can see deep into the clear blue water. You can feel the water touching your skin and supporting your body. You can hear the splashing of minnows in the distance. You smell the water's clean scent.

Or you might imagine sitting next to a stream. Your feet dangle in the cool rush of water. You can see and hear the water splashing against the rocks. You feel its mist touching your skin. It smells so refreshing.

Or you might picture walking through the mist or rain. Far in the distance you can see the soft clouds overhead. Gentle drops touch your skin. You can hear the rain as it hits the ground. And you notice how clean the rain makes the air smell.

For the next minute or so let yourself enjoy a daydream involving water. Involve all of your senses.

[PAUSE 1 MINUTE]

Gently let go of what you are attending to.

We are ready to move on.

There is more to discover in our special relaxing place. Imagine you discover a special relaxing building or house. It can be anything.

You might imagine yourself in a peaceful forest cabin. You can see the wood walls and fireplace. You can hear the wind outside and crackling fire. You can feel the heat of the fire touching your skin, and you can smell the soothing odor of burning logs.

Or you might think of a childhood room. What did it look like? Did you have anything special on the walls? Maybe you can smell food cooking in the distance or hear pets scampering underfoot. What is touching your skin?

Or you might imagine a church or temple, with its majestic and reassuring arches. You can hear the soft sound of music in the background or smell flowers or incense. As you sit, you can feel the firm chair holding you.

For the next minute or so let yourself enjoy a daydream in a peaceful indoor setting. Involve all of your senses.

(continued)

TABLE 3.12   *(continued)*

[PAUSE 1 MINUTE]

Gently let go of what you are attending to.

And now, for a moment, think about the journey we have just taken. What part was most relaxing? What part did you enjoy? Did you like traveling? An outdoor nature setting? The water theme? Or the relaxing building or house? Which part of your journey did you enjoy most?

[FOR TAPE PRESENTATION, SKIP TO DRESS REHEARSAL.]

Of course, there are many possible daydreams you could have for each.

[PRESENT SENSE IMAGERY LIST.]

What theme do you want?

[CLIENT PICKS THEME, OR GROUP NOMINATES AND VOTES ON ONE THEME THAT INSTRUCTOR WILL USE IN GROUP EXERCISE.]

Sometimes people pick a daydream theme that runs into problems. It might seem fine at first but has a hidden booby trap within. For example, you might want to think of the lake you visited as a child, not realizing you nearly drowned in the lake. This painful thought might arise unexpectedly in your daydream and spoil your relaxation. Can you think of any hidden problems in your theme?

[IF PROBLEMS ARE MENTIONED, PICK ANOTHER THEME.]

Now we need to paint the details for your theme. What might you see? What might you hear or feel touching your skin? What might you smell that is relaxing? Let's see if we can think of some ideas while I write them down.

[ASK CLIENT FOR AT LEAST 4 OR 5 SENSE DETAILS FOR EACH CATEGORY: WHAT IS SEEN, HEARD, FELT, AND SMELLED. WRITE THEM DOWN ON YOUR SENSE IMAGERY WORKSHEET. FOR GROUP, ASK GROUP MEMBERS TO NOMINATE SENSE DETAILS FOR NOMINATED THEME. INCLUDE NO MORE THAN FOUR FOR EACH.]

DRESS REHEARSAL

We are now ready to try your daydream.

[PROCEED WITH A DISENGAGEMENT COUNTDOWN.]

Let yourself settle into a peaceful state of relaxation.

TABLE 3.12 *(continued)*

As you relax, I will begin to count backward, from 5 to 1. With every count, let yourself sink into a pleasant state of relaxation, far from the concerns of the world.

[PAUSE]

Five.

You begin to settle into a state of relaxation, letting go of the concerns of the day. There is nothing you have to do.

Four.

The world becomes more and more distant, as you let go and relax. You feel very safe and comfortable.

Three.

Let yourself sink deeper and deeper into relaxation. You notice your breathing become more slow and even. You begin to feel heavy and relaxed.

Two.

You sink farther and farther away from the concerns of the world. You become more and more relaxed, as if you were sinking into the world of sleep and dreams.

And one.

We are now ready to begin our special relaxing daydream. Let's return to the part of our relaxing journey you enjoyed the most. Think of what it was like. Involve all of your senses.

[HERE THE TRAINER PRESENTS A SERIES OF SENSE SUGGESTIONS DRAWN FROM CLIENT'S LIST. TRAINER SUGGESTS ONE FROM EACH OF THE FOUR CATEGORIES, UNTIL A TOTAL OF THREE OR FOUR SUGGESTIONS IS EVENTU-ALLY PRESENTED FROM EACH CATEGORY. FOR EXAMPLE, TRAINER SAYS: "YOU SEE THE BLUE SKY (WHAT YOU SEE) . . . YOU HEAR THE WIND IN THE TREES . . . YOU FEEL THE WARM SUN ON YOUR SKIN . . . YOU HEAR BIRDS IN THE DISTANCE (NOW ONE SUGGESTION HAS BEEN PRESENTED FROM EACH CATEGORY). . . . YOU SEE THE TREES FAR IN THE DIS-TANCE . . . HEAR THE BIRDS SINGING QUIETLY . . . FEEL THE TOUCH OF SPRING MIST . . . AND SMELL THE FRESH SCENT OF FLOW-ERS . . . CLOUDS FLOAT GENTLY OVERHEAD . . . THE TREES RUSTLE IN THE WIND . . . THE WIND TOUCHES YOUR SKIN . . . THE FRAGRANCE OF FLOWERS IS SO PEACEFUL" (NOW THREE SUGGESTIONS HAVE BEEN PRESENTED FROM EACH CATEGORY.)]

Now, for the next 10 minutes let yourself enjoy your relaxing fantasy. Involve all of your senses.

(continued)

TABLE 3.12   *(continued)*

[PAUSE 10 MINUTES]

Gently let go of what you are attending to. We have finished our daydream exercise. Gently open your eyes. And take a deep breath and stretch. How did that go?

[PROCESS EXERCISE, ADDING MODIFICATIONS IF PROBLEMS AROSE.]

For this week, you are to practice 15 minutes of your daydream fantasy each day. Your fantasy may change, but stay with the general theme you have selected so that it can grow on you. And before each session, do a few minutes of squeezing, stretching, or breathing as preparation.

Sense Imagery List

Travel	Outdoor/ Nature	Water	Indoor
Rowboat	Forest	Hot tub	Cabin
Sailboat	Plain	Rain	Childhood
Canoe	Garden	Mist	home
Balloon	Mountaintop	On the ocean	Skyscraper
Rocket ship	Valley	beach	penthouse
Just floating	Park	In a pond	House of
Hang gliding	Nature trail	On the lake	dreams
Automobile	Desert	Under a	Special room
Train	Glacier	waterfall	Chapel
Submarine	Snow-covered	By the river	Church
Horse	landscape	Floating down	Synagog
	The moon at	the river	
	night		

TABLE 3.12 *(continued)*

SENSE IMAGERY WORKSHEET

Imagery theme:

What is seen?

What is heard?

What is felt touching the skin?

What fragrances are smelled?

TABLE 3.13   Script for Insight Imagery

(Words that are in **boldface** or [BRACKETED] are special instructions to trainers. These words are not to be read or spoken to clients.)

RATIONALE/EXPLANATION

In this exercise we are going to learn to relax with a special type of imagery. Imagery can be a way of experiencing calm and peace. Before we begin, I would like to share with you an interesting and unusual little list. Over the years, researchers have been asking people what thoughts and ideas help them relax, what thoughts and ideas help create calm and peace. Of course, different people find different ideas relaxing. What may be a source of calm and peace for you may not be a source of calm and peace to other people.

Here's a list of what the researchers found.

Let's take a look at these phrases. Are there any that you believe? Maybe some phrases that work for you are not on this list.

[DISTRIBUTE R-BELIEFS INVENTORY.]

I want to reassure you that this is not a quiz. I will not be giving you a test later on. As you can see from this list, many different types of ideas can be sources of calm and peace for different people.

And now, let's put this list aside.

We are ready to begin with our exercise.

In this imagery we will enjoy a relaxing story in which you might learn more about yourself and relaxation. We took a look at some thoughts and ideas that can be a source of calm and peace. In this exercise we will discover that imagery can also be a way of experiencing calm and peace.

This exercise has two parts. First, we will try a little sample imagery, just to get in the proper state of mind. This can give you an idea of what imagery is all about, and help you come up with some ideas of what you want in your imagery.

Then we will spend about 10 minutes actually doing imagery, using the details you like best.

First, make sure you are seated upright in a comfortable position. Are your feet resting comfortably on the floor? Close your eyes, and relax.

[PAUSE ABOUT 30 SECONDS FOR CLIENT OR GROUP TO RELAX.]

DEMONSTRATION

First we try a brief sample image, to get ready.

This image is actually a story of a journey. In it you go to a special place, one that has a message of calm and peace for you.

TABLE 3.13 *(continued)*

There is nothing for you to do or think about. Simply relax and enjoy the journey.

Imagine you are traveling a long distance. Perhaps you are in a boat, a train, or even a balloon; it doesn't matter. You see many wonderful things coming and going. The sky. The scenery outside. You can feel the sun and fresh air. You can hear the wind and smell the fresh fragrance of trees.

[PAUSE]

You come to the end of your journey. It is an outdoor nature setting.

[PAUSE]

It is a wonderful and beautiful place, filled with mystery and wonder.

You can see green all around—trees, grass, flowers. The sky above is a clear blue. You can feel a gentle breeze against your skin.

And the warm sun.
You hear the wind blowing through the trees or grass.
Perhaps you hear the song of a distant bird.
It is a wonderful and relaxing place.
And in this place you discover a clear pond.

Its surface is very still, like a perfect mirror that reflects the blue sky and clouds above. In the distance you notice a person walking, someone who is very wise. This can be a religious leader, a philosopher, teacher, or someone in your life.

This setting has a special message for you. It is a special message of calm, peace, and happiness. This message can come to you in many ways. Perhaps the message will appear reflected in the surface of the pond. Perhaps the person in the distance has a message to give you. The message can be anything. It can even be something as simple as your beautiful surroundings, which create feelings of calm, peace, and happiness.

And there is absolutely nothing you have to do.

Simply and calmly attend to this relaxing setting without trying to figure anything out. Let it reveal its message to you in whatever way it wants.

If thoughts come to mind, that's fine. Simply and gently put them aside, and continue attending.

If you find yourself starting to figure things out, that's fine. Simply put your thoughts aside and calmly attend to the setting. Enjoy it and attend to what it has to say to you. That is all you need to do.

(continued)

TABLE 3.13 *(continued)*

[WAIT 1 MINUTE]

Gently let go of what you are thinking of.

[PAUSE]

We are ready to consider your imagery story.

What was it like? What type of theme do you want?

[WAIT FOR ANSWER. RECORD ON WORKSHEET.]

Sometimes people pick a daydream theme that runs into problems. It might seem fine at first, but it has a hidden booby trap within. For example, you might want to think of the lake you visited as a child, not realizing you nearly drowned in the lake. This painful thought might arise unexpectedly in your daydream and spoil your relaxation. Can you think of any hidden problems in your theme?

[IF PROBLEMS ARE MENTIONED, PICK ANOTHER THEME.]

[IN GROUP EXERCISE, PAUSE. GROUP SELECTS SPECIFICS OF THEME AND IMAGERY DETAILS: THE NATURE OF THE MESSAGE OF "CALM AND PEACE" AND HOW AND WHERE IT APPEARS.]

Now we need to paint the details for your theme. What might you see? What might you hear or feel touching your skin? What might you smell that is relaxing? Let's see if we can think of some ideas while I write them down.

[ASK CLIENT FOR AT LEAST 4 OR 5 SENSE DETAILS FOR EACH CATEGORY: WHAT IS SEEN, HEARD, FELT, AND SMELLED. WRITE THEM DOWN ON YOUR INSIGHT IMAGERY WORKSHEET. FOR GROUP, ASK GROUP MEMBERS TO NOMINATE SENSE DETAILS FOR NOMINATED THEME. INCLUDE NO MORE THAN FOUR FOR EACH.]

Finally, in your fantasy story, how do you want your message of calm, peace, and happiness to appear? There is no need to tell me your answer. This is just for you. Your message can appear in many ways. Sometimes the message is nothing more than the beautiful setting itself. Maybe it is reflected in a pond. Perhaps a wise person in your image whispers the message to you. How do you want it to appear? It is okay to leave this question unanswered and simply enjoy the imagery.

[DO NOT RECORD CLIENT'S RESPONSE TO THIS FINAL INQUIRY. THIS IS VERY PERSONAL, FOR THE CLIENT ONLY.]

TABLE 3.13 *(continued)*

DRESS REHEARSAL

Imagine _____ [NAME CLIENT'S OR GROUP'S THEME].

Let yourself become more and more relaxed. Involve all of your senses.

[HERE TRAINER PRESENTS A SERIES OF SENSE SUGGESTIONS DRAWN FROM CLIENT'S LIST. TRAINER SUGGESTS ONE FROM EACH OF THE FOUR CATEGO-RIES, UNTIL A TOTAL OF THREE OR FOUR SUGGESTIONS IS EVENTUALLY PRESENTED FROM EACH CATEGORY. FOR EXAMPLE, TRAINER SAYS: "YOU SEE THE BLUE SKY (WHAT YOU SEE) . . . YOU HEAR THE WIND IN THE TREES . . . YOU FEEL THE WARM SUN ON YOUR SKIN . . . YOU HEAR BIRDS IN THE DISTANCE (NOW ONE SUGGESTION HAS BEEN PRESENTED FROM EACH CATE-GORY). . . . YOU SEE THE TREES FAR IN THE DISTANCE . . . HEAR THE BIRDS SINGING QUIETLY . . . FEEL THE TOUCH OF SPRING MIST . . . AND SMELL THE FRESH SCENT OF FLOWERS. . . . CLOUDS FLOAT GENTLY OVERHEAD . . . THE TREES RUSTLE IN THE WIND . . . THE WIND TOUCHES YOUR SKIN . . . THE FRAGRANCE OF FLOWERS IS SO PEACEFUL" (NOW THREE SUGGESTIONS HAVE BEEN PRESENTED FROM EACH CATEGORY.)]

Now, for the next 10 minutes let yourself enjoy your relaxing imagery. Involve all of your senses.

[PAUSE 10 MINUTES]

Gently let go of what you are attending to. We have finished our daydream exercise. Gently open your eyes. And take a deep breath and stretch. How did that go?

[PROCESS EXERCISE, ADDING MODIFICATIONS IF PROBLEMS AROSE.]

For this week, you are to practice 15 minutes of your daydream fantasy each day. Your fantasy may change, but stay with the general theme you have selected so that it can grow on you. And before each session, do a few minutes of squeezing, stretching, or breathing as preparation.

(continued)

TABLE 3.13 *(continued)*

INSIGHT IMAGERY WORKSHEET

Imagery theme:

What is seen?

What is heard?

What is felt touching the skin?

What fragrances are smelled?

APPROACH 6: MEDITATION

Meditation is perhaps the most challenging form of relaxation. Of all techniques, it is the most passive and focused. Indeed, the instructions for meditation are essentially instructions to "sustain passive simple focusing" and do nothing else. Specifically, all forms of meditation involve continuously attending to an utterly singular stimulus or to the moment-to-moment flow of all stimuli. I introduce eight approaches to meditation (Table 3.14), seven associated with the seven families of relaxation activities (see *ABC Relaxation Theory*).

Of these, I have found rocking meditation to be the easiest and most readily practiced; the remaining are about equally challenging. Contrary to the nearly universal preference among Western meditation instructors for mantra meditation, I find this approach no easier than others.

My research suggests that meditation evokes Mental Quiet and, like yoga and breathing, Strength and Awareness, Joy, Love and Thankfulness, and Prayerfulness. My clinical experience suggests that at times it fosters Disengagement (as when one becomes "fully aware and focused" while "withdrawing from distraction").

Researchers have been a bit confused about the application of meditation. The specificity model considers meditation to be cognitive (Davidson & Schwartz, 1976). Yet meditation appears to have some impact on somatic symptoms (Lehrer, Carr, Sargunaraj, & Woolfolk, 1994). If we were to list the claimed applications of meditation, they would include every application listed for every other technique. The most widely practiced and researched form of meditation in America, transcendental meditation (TM), has added to the confusion. TM's Maharhishi International

TABLE 3.14   Eight Approaches to Meditation

Relaxation Family	Related Meditation
Somatic/emotion	Somatic sensation—meditation on physical sensations of relaxation
Breathing	Breath meditation
Movement/posture	Movement—Rocking meditation
Internal cognitive (vocal/auditory)	Mantra meditation
Internal cognitive (visual)	Meditation on a simple mental image
External (vocal/auditory)	Meditation on a simple sound (chant, etc.)
External (visual)	Meditation on a visual stimulus (candle)
	Mindfulness meditation

University, fully accredited and staffed by licensed doctoral-level professionals, makes claims not made for any other formal approach to relaxation. TM is "proven" to increase IQ, cure illness, and evoke paranormal and superhuman powers, including the power to levitate, become invisible, and directly access and manipulate reality itself at the quantum level (Smith, 1990). Given this culture of overstatement, I chose not to make any tabular claims for meditation. I invite practitioners to try meditation with an open mind and with modest expectations.

Meditation is a difficult technique, one perhaps best attempted after mastering another form of relaxation as preparation. It is an approach (with the possible exception of rocking meditation or short, 5-minute "mini-meditations") not appropriate for individuals who have difficulty concentrating, are easily distracted, or need a highly structured and familiar training format. Caution should be taken when teaching meditation to individuals who may have a strong irrational religion-based opposition to meditation.

In presenting meditation, speak softly, simply, and clearly. Avoid all color and inflection, but do not make your voice boring and monotonous. Use short, clear sentences. Cultivate a tone of voice that is alert and clear.

Step 1: Explanation and Rationale

I try to present meditation in a way consistent with the utter simplicity of the technique. For a rationale, I just present the overall instructions, "Attend to a simple stimulus. Return attention after every distraction." Warn clients that distractions are not only normal but part of the process of learning meditation.

Steps 2 and 3: Demonstration, Dress Rehearsal

I then present 90-second demonstrations of seven modalities of meditation, ending with mindfulness, and invite clients to continue for 3 minutes on their preferred technique. See Table 3.15 for a complete script.

Steps 4 and 5: Checking and Modification

Distractions

Distraction is perhaps the universal experience of meditation, for beginners and advanced practitioners alike. All kinds of thoughts may come to mind—memories, plans for the day, emotions, images, physical sensations, sounds from the outside, and so on. Many beginners have the mistaken belief that to practice correctly somehow requires avid, unwavering concentration, as if meditation were akin to playing a video game (where a second's lapse of attention can lose millions of points). In fact, distraction is a normal part of meditation. Indeed, one must be distracted in order to develop in meditation.

The goal of meditation is not so much to concentrate the mind as it is to consistently and calmly return attention to a focal object after every task. This may happen hundreds of times a session. However, one returns attention as calmly and restfully as possible. It is only through such opportunities to *return* attention that one gradually trains oneself to focus in meditation.

I invite trainees to consider the following two meditators, meditating on the word *one*. Both show exactly the same number of distractions; the second is dealing with them properly while the first is not:

"One . . . One . . . One . . . Hmmm, I want a hamburger. Darn it! I got distracted. I must concentrate better! DAMMIT! ONE! . . . ONE! . . . ONE! . . . "

"One . . . One . . . One . . . Hmmm, I want a hamburger. Oops, One . . . One . . . One . . . "

There are meditative and unmeditative ways of dealing with distraction. Some meditative reactions include the following:

"No problem . . . easily return."

"I'm distracted. That's okay, a part of meditation. Gently return."

"My mind wandered again. How interesting. Back to meditation."

"Oh, hello, distraction. I can spend time with you later, after my meditation. Good-bye."

Some unmeditative responses include

"My mind wandered. I'll never meditate. I feel so frustrated."

"Oh, what an important thought about my work problem. I have to think about it or my problem won't get solved."

"Hmmm, this distraction's fun. I'll just stay with it. This is just as good as meditating."

Several seasoned meditation instructors have some helpful descriptions of this easy, permissive way of dealing with distraction in meditation. Larence LeShan (1974) says:

> Give yourself permission to make constant slips from the directions. You will make them anyway and will be much more comfortable—and get along better with this exercise—if you give yourself permission in advance. Treat yourself as if you were a much-loved child that an adult was trying to keep walking on a narrow sidewalk. The child is full of energy and keeps running off to the fields on each side to pick flowers, feel the grass, climb a tree. Each time you are aware of the child leaving the path, you say in effect, "Oh, that's how children are. Okay, honey, back to the sidewalk," and bring yourself gently but firmly and alertly back to just looking. Again and again you will suddenly notice that you are thinking about something else or translating your perception into words or something of the sort. Each time, you should say the equivalent of "Oh, that's where I am now; back to the work." (p. 54)

Pat Carrington, a friend of mine and fellow meditation instructor, says:

> When meditating never *force* thoughts out of your mind. All kinds of thoughts may drift through your mind while you are meditating. Treat these thoughts just as you would treat clouds drifting across the sky. You don't push the clouds away—but you don't hold onto them either. You just watch them come and go. It's the same with thoughts during meditation, you just watch them, and then when it feels comfortable to do so, go back. (p. 25)

Elsewhere, Carrington advises against struggling against intruding thoughts when meditating. Such distractions are a natural part of everyone's meditative experience. Indeed they can be a sign that meditation is working. She suggests greeting distracting thoughts

> as you would a friend whom you like but with whom you do not have time to talk right now. Imagine that you are letting this friend walk alongside you, but you are not becoming involved in conversation with him/her. In other words, flow *with* the thoughts that turn up during meditation and allow them full play, but do not cling to them. (p. 20)

Some liken distraction to silt at the bottom of a cool and quiet pond. This silt, when stirred, can cloud the waters. The return action of meditation is a way of clearing the mind of potential future distraction. Each meditative return is like a cleaning sweep along the bottom of the pond. Somewhat less poetically, by permitting distractions to come and go we may be releasing or discharging subtle inner tensions that might cloud meditation.

The Problem of Mindfulness

Mindfulness meditation can be difficult to describe. I find it best to start with very simple and somewhat poetic instructions (as in the script in Table 3.15) and then present elaborations as problems arise. In mindfulness meditation, the object is not to attend to a preselected stimulus. Instead, one quietly attends to, notes, and lets go of every stimulus that enters awareness—every thought, feeling, sensation, sound, idea, and so on. One does not try to figure out, think about, push away, or do anything with the thoughts, feelings, and sensations experienced. Simply let each stimulus come and go and wait for the next stimulus. The mindful meditator is nothing more than a neutral observer, viewing the world as it is, uncolored by reactions, judgments, and evaluations.

Mindfulness meditation is just about impossible to explain logically. It can be useful to think of several images, for example, that of sitting beside a quietly flowing stream. A variety of unexpected objects slowly and continuously floats by. A piece of wood comes into sight and then floats away. Then a patch of leaves. An then a floating seed. In mindfulness meditation, treat every thought, feeling, and sensation as something that drifts into view on its own. The task is utterly simple: acknowledge that it is there ("Oh, a thought . . . this is interesting") and let it drift away after a few seconds. Calmly wait until something else floats into view.

Or one might think of the image of calmly resting in a tent in the evening woods. There is nothing to do or figure out; it is peaceful and secure. Sounds come and go, for example, the rush of the wind. Listen, without thinking or trying to figure things out, and quietly return to listening once again. The trees smell so refreshing. Note this and return to a peacefully quiet and attentive stance. A bird sings far in the distance. One thinks, "Oh, the sound of a bird," and returns to quietly listening again. In other words, all the mindful meditator does is note each sensation, let go of what he or she is sensing, and continue attending.

Many people try to do too much with mindfulness meditation. One doesn't have to figure out the connections between each of the stimuli; often there will be none. The task is not to look for deeper understandings. There is no need to attend to any thought, feeling, or sensation for any length of time. Indeed, one should dwell on any particular "floating object" or "sound of the night" for only several seconds—about the time it takes a real-life leaf to float in and out of sight on a stream or the time it takes a gentle gust of wind to blow and settle into silence. And in mindfulness meditation one doesn't have to be concerned about distractions. Each time one is distracted, the meditator notes it as yet another passing stimulus ("Ah, a distraction—how interesting"), lets go of it, and gently and easily returns to attending to whatever stimuli may drift past awareness.

The following are suggestions for enhancing meditation:

• Do not teach meditation by itself. Precede with any other relaxation exercise. I recommend a 20-minute premeditation "warm-up" consisting of stretching and breathing exercises.
• Clients who find it difficult to attend to a simple meditative focus may benefit from combined meditations, for example, rocking and breathing or breathing and mantra meditation.
• Beginners may benefit from brief meditations, 5–10 minutes in length.
• Practice in a simple, meditative setting, suggestive of Mental Quiet, Mental Relaxation, Strength and Awareness, and Prayerfulness.

TABLE 3.15   Script for Meditation

(Words that are in **boldface** or [BRACKETED] are special instructions to trainers. These words are not to be read or spoken to clients.)

RATIONALE

[PREPARATION: BRING A CANDLE AND A BELL OR CHIME.]

Meditation is a very simple exercise. In fact, the instructions can be said in two sentences: Calmly attend to a simple stimulus. Calmly return your attention after every distraction . . . again and again and again. In this exercise we will try seven meditations and end with an approach called mindfulness. You will have a chance to select which work best for you. One of our meditations involves a candle, which I will now light.

[LIGHT CANDLE.]

DEMONSTRATION

Body Sense Meditation

Let's begin by closing our eyes. Make sure you are seated comfortably in an upright position. Your feet should be flat on the floor.

TABLE 3.15 *(continued)*

[PAUSE]

For the next minute or so, let go of the concerns of the day. This time is for you alone. There is nothing you have to do or figure out.

[PAUSE]

Let go of any tensions you might feel. And relax.

[PAUSE]

How does your body feel as you begin to relax? Warm? Sinking? Heavy? Perhaps you notice a warm glow in your abdomen, like the good feeling from drinking hot chocolate or soup.

[PAUSE]

For the next minute or so, simply let go of tension and quietly attend to how your body feels. Whenever you start thinking about what you are doing, simply let go of these thoughts and return to attending to how your relaxing body feels.

[PAUSE 45 SECONDS.]

Rocking Meditation

We are ready to move on. Think of all the times in life you have found the gentle movement of *rocking* very calm and soothing. You might be on a rowboat in a lake, gently bobbing back and forth as waves gently lap against you. Perhaps you are in a rocking chair on a porch. You are at peace. Nothing is on your mind. You gently rock back and forth, again and again. Perhaps you are resting on a hammock, swinging very gently. You might even be rocking a small child in your arms. There is indeed something very soothing and meditative about simple rocking.

At this time let yourself begin to rock back and forth in your chair.

[PAUSE]

Let each movement become more and more gentle and easy. Let yourself rock effortlessly. Let your body move on its own, in its own way, at its own speed. All you have to do is simply attend.

[PAUSE]

(continued)

TABLE 3.15 *(continued)*

Let each movement become more and more subtle so that someone watching would barely notice you are rocking. For the next minute or so, quietly attend to gentle and silent rocking.

[PAUSE 90 SECONDS]

Gently let go of what you are attending to. Meditation is very simple. If your mind wandered, that's OK. If you are distracted, that's OK.

Breathing Meditation

We move on. Take in a full breath, and relax. Let your breathing continue on its own in a way that is free and easy. There is nothing you have to so. Simply attend to the flow of breath, in and out. And return your attention whenever your mind wanders or is distracted.

[PAUSE 90 SECONDS]

Mantra Meditation

Gently let go of what you are attending to. Let a relaxing word, perhaps the word *peace*, come to you like an echo in the distance. Let the word go over and over and over, at its own pace and volume.

The word doesn't have to go with your breath. Simply attend as the word quietly and easily goes over and over. When your mind wanders or you are distracted, that's OK. Simply return.

[PAUSE 90 SECONDS]

Meditation on a Visual Image

Gently let go of what you are attending to. With your eyes closed, think of the image of a simple spot of light, a candle flame, or a star.

And calmly attend.

And calmly return after every distraction.

TABLE 3.15 *(continued)*

[PAUSE 90 SECONDS]

Meditation on an External Image

Gently let go of what you are attending to. Slowly open your eyes halfway. Easily gaze on the candle in front of you. Whenever your mind wanders, gently return.

[PAUSE 90 SECONDS]

Meditation on a Sound

And now, quietly listen to this sound as it rings and dissolves into silence.

[RING CHIME OR BELL ONCE. WAIT FOR 1 MINUTE.]

Mindfulness Meditation

And gently let go of what you are attending to. If you wish, open your eyes.

The world is alive with sounds and sights and sensations.

You are a mirror.

Quietly reflect what passes by. There is no reason to think about anything.

[PAUSE]

With your eyes closed and without thinking about anything, what do you notice about you? What sound or sight or sensation comes to you?

[PAUSE]

Whenever you notice something, fine. Gently name it, put it aside, and continue attending with an open mind until you notice something else.

[PAUSE]

When you notice something again, just quietly name it, put it aside, and resume attending.

(continued)

TABLE 3.15   *(continued)*

You are a neutral observer, waiting very calmly and peacefully
. . . doing nothing but noting what comes to mind.

Each moment comes and goes. The river of time slowly passes by.

[PAUSE 90 SECONDS; RING CHIME.]

And now gently let go of what you are attending to. We have explored these meditations:

Attending to your body as it relaxes.

Gently rocking.

The flow of breath, in and out.

Attending to the word *peace* as it goes over and over.

Attending to a spot of light with your eyes closed.

A candle flame.

The sound of a chime.

We concluded by becoming neutral observers, mirrors reflecting the coming and going of all stimuli.

Which one, if any, did you like best?

[PAUSE 15 SECONDS]

DRESS REHEARSAL

For the next few minutes, quietly attend to the one meditation you liked best.

Your body relaxes . . . rocking . . . breathing . . . the word *peace* . . . a spot of light . . . a candle flame . . . a chime . . . the coming and going of the moment.

Quietly attend, and return your attention after every distraction . . . again and again and again.

[PAUSE 3 MINUTES]

Quietly let go of what you are attending to. Slowly open your eyes all the way. Take a deep breath and stretch. This completes our meditation exercise.

TABLE 3.15 *(continued)*

Here is a list of the types of meditation we have tried. Which do you want to be your meditation?

[PRESENT MEDITATION SELECTION CHART.]

MEDITATION SELECTION CHART

_____ Meditation on body relaxing

_____ Rocking meditation

_____ Breathing meditation

_____ Meditation on "peace" or a relaxing word or syllable (name word or syllable: _____)

_____ Meditation on a simple mental image (name: _____)

_____ Meditation on a candle

_____ Meditation on the sound of a bell, or other sounds

_____ Being like a mirror, a neutral observer; mindfulness meditation

PRACTICING RELAXATION SPEECH PATTERNS

It is useful to emphasize that voice volume, speed, and inflection can have a profound impact on the success of relaxation training. Indeed, when training therapists to deploy a "voice" appropriate to a technique, I have them practice on a phone book. The voice quality alone should be sufficient to suggest the quality of relaxation associated with a technique. The following are key differences among techniques.

PMR

"Tense up" talk should be relatively loud and tense, as if you were a gym coach urging your students to put forth more effort. "Let go" talk should communicate letting go. The first "let go" phrase (of the four) should be spoken with a sigh, almost as if you were letting go—"And let go-o-o-o." The remaining phrases should be spoken slowly and softly, in a rather gentle, monotonous, and uninteresting monotone, something like a tape recording that has been deliberately slowed or like the voice of someone who is dozing off.

Autogenic Training

Speak in a slow monotone, showing little inflection and color.

Breathing Exercises

Pattern instructions with your own inhalations and exhalations. In addition, add a touch of "breathiness" to your speech, increasing the flow of air as you speak each word. The voice should be calm, refreshed, and alert.

Yoga Stretching

Speak slowly, suggesting the act of slowly stretching and unstretching. Elongate vowels ("Sloooowly stretch"). Speak as if you were stretching yourself. The voice should be calm, refreshed, and alert.

Imagery

Disengaging talk should be quiet and rather monotonous. Engaging talk should be a bit more "colorful," with inflections corresponding to key story phrases. Such engaging talk is not unlike the storytelling voice one might employ in telling an interesting story to a child.

Meditation

Speak softly, simply, and clearly. Avoid all color and inflection, but do not make your voice boring and monotonous. Use short, clear sentences.

In rehearsing relaxation voice quality, I have trainees read typical excerpts from major techniques (Table 3.16 at the end of the chapter), interrupting and coaching when appropriate. With a group of trainees, it can be very effective to have students provide feedback to each other.

TROUBLESHOOTING

The Problem of N-States

Any form of relaxation can evoke unwanted or aversive states of mind. Such N-States (negative states) can include physical sensations, negative emotions, and worry. Their sources are many. Some N-States reflect how one appraises relaxation:

Resistance to Letting Go

In everyday life we accomplish our tasks through planning and effort; in relaxation, we must let go of planning and effort in order to achieve greater simplicity of focus. A beginning relaxer can find this basic shift difficult, feeling that the task of letting go in order to achieve the possible benefits of relaxation is impossible.

Fears over "Losing Control"

A relaxer may fear the task of letting go and mistakenly think it means "going crazy," "becoming sick," and so on.

Concerns about Reduced Personal Efficacy

Clients may fear relaxation will contribute to "laziness," "giving up," or reduced ability to work or perform at peak efficiency.

Negative Appraisal of R-States

Clients may not be familiar with many of the R-States we have previously identified, including physiological signs of reduced arousal (e.g., increased blood flow to the extremities, reduced breathing and heart rate), symptom reduction, feelings of somatic and cognitive tension relief, as well as disengagement and mental quiet. Not knowing such experiences are a normal part of relaxation, clients may find them threatening and fear becoming ill, going "crazy," and so on.

Previous Aversive Experiences with Relaxation

An occasional client may have had an aversive or even traumatic experience related to relaxation. Clients have been sexually harassed by hypnotists, manipulated and threatened by yoga instructors, lied to by meditation gurus, taught ineptly by coercive PMR trainers, or simply taught that relaxation is "weird and occult." Past negative experiences with relaxation can limit a client's willingness to attempt relaxation again and stir distress in the course of relaxation training.

Negative Associations to Relaxation Techniques

A relaxation technique may remind a client of a negative experience that has nothing to do with the technique itself. For example, a client may relax with imagery that involves an ocean beach, only to remember a painful childhood sunburn. Such relaxation booby traps are most common when techniques are mechanically imposed on clients with little attempt to individualize.

Other forms of N-States reflect secondary processes set into motion through sustained passive simple focus.

Increased Sensitivity

One consequence of all relaxation training is the reduction of potentially distracting internal and external stimuli. In the quiet of a practice session, a relaxer may simply notice subtle sources of stimuli that ordinarily go undetected. He or she may be aware of breathing, heart rate, underlying emotional state, and so on. Unprepared, a client may appraise such experiences as threats.

Disengagement, Disorientation, and Depersonalization

Through disengagement, the relaxer pulls away from and becomes less aware of the outside world. In relaxation this contributes to singular focus of a restricted stimulus by minimizing distraction. However, if a relaxer resumes everyday activities while remaining disengaged, he or she may experience disruptive depersonalization or disorientation.

Reduction of Defensive Barriers

Relaxation can reduce defensive efforts to deny or ignore threatening thoughts and feelings. For a skilled psychotherapist, the resulting emergence of threatening material can provide a basis for treatment. However, such uncovered material can interfere with the course of relaxation if not properly managed.

Reductions in Critical Thinking and Reality Testing

As one relaxes, one reduces deliberate efforts at analysis and control, including critical and analytic thinking. In some contexts this can contribute to enjoyment, as when one temporarily suspends disbelief and becomes absorbed in a movie or novel. However, lessened critical thinking and reality testing may make one more susceptible to troublesome thoughts and fantasies that might arise in relaxation. For example, in the course of a day's events a client may casually wonder: "Sometimes I feel like I am floating in relaxation. Do I really float?" He or she may ordinarily appraise such a feeling reasonably; "Of course, I am not really floating; I'm just experiencing a relaxation effect." However, if such a thought were to arise in deep relaxation, rational and reality-based assessment has decreased. Our client may well "suspend disbelief," actually believe he or she is levitating, and experience distress.

Hyperventilation/Hypoventilation

We have seen that changes in breathing in relaxation can result in decreased or increased blood levels of carbon dioxide (CO_2). Such hyper- or hypoventilation can lead to aversive subjective states, including dizziness and anxiety.

Presumed Shifts in Brain Functioning

As relaxation deepens, parts of the brain, perhaps the cerebral cortex, may become relatively less active. Other parts, perhaps those less active in active daily life, become relatively more active. This could result in increased spontaneous, wakeful dreamlike activity, including vivid imagery, novel or intense emotional states, changes in body image (sensations of floating, changing size), and even felt paranormal phenomena.

Managing N-States in Relaxation

It is often sufficient to explain that students of relaxation, like students of any other discipline, whether sports, dance, or others, experience "ups and downs." Such cycles are a natural part of growth and movement (*see* my book *ABC Relaxation Theory*). The very process of "going deeper" in a session can unearth distractions and problems. In the relaxation session proper, the response to such nonspecific distractions is generally to resume practice. This, indeed, is how skill at relaxation develops. However, if problems persist, or are disruptive beyond the practice session, a trainer might experiment with the following modifications:

1. Shorten an exercise.
2. Practice an exercise with less vigor (especially important for physical approaches).
3. Precede an exercise (especially mental) with 5 to 10 minutes of preferred physical relaxation exercises as warm-up.
4. Select less focused or passive exercises in the chosen domain. For example, instead of meditating on one's breath, a client might attempt diaphragmatic breathing.
5. Attempt exercises from a different domain.
6. Provide greater structure perhaps by shortening pauses and periods of silence and instead continuing instructional "patter."
7. Increase exercise complexity by introducing elements of several exercises.
8. Revise an exercise, deleting any elements that trigger distressing associations.
9. Introduce phrases of encouragement and support.
10. Supplement exercise with music or tapes of nature sounds.
11. Increase extraneous stimulation (turn up lights, open the windows, select a familiar and somewhat complex relaxation environment, practice in an upright seated position, practice standing up).
12. Practice in a group.
13. Take a break or vacation from professional relaxation and emphasize familiar casual approaches not likely to cause problems.
14. In instructions, remove phrases suggestive of Disengagement.
15. In instructions, emphasize phrases suggestive of specific effects (symptom reduction, tension relief, positive feelings).

If relaxation-induced distress persists, professional psychotherapy may be advised.

Drowsiness and Sleep

Nearly everyone who has learned a relaxation technique has fallen asleep from time to time. Clients often wonder if drowsiness and sleep are normal and are concerned about what to do if they become a problem. The R-State Sleepiness is a normal part of most relaxation, particularly cognitive approaches and PMR. However, Sleepiness can be a needless distraction if it is caused by factors unrelated to relaxation. Some of these factors are listed below.

Inability to Differentiate Relaxation from Sleep

The beginning practitioner of relaxation often has a vague, undifferentiated perspective of the nature of relaxation. Just as a beginning chef may see all oriental cuisines as the same, a novice relaxer may think of all relaxation techniques as different approaches to napping. Similarly, a beginning relaxer may find it difficult to differentiate between the effects we have just outlined and may see all in terms of the one relaxation experience he or she knows well, falling asleep.

Inability to Differentiate Disengagement from Sleep

Because feelings of Disengagement often precede normal sleep, clients may often think they are falling asleep when Disengaging from distracting stimuli in relaxation. In relaxation, unlike sleep, Disengagement is accompanied by maintained attention on a simple stimulus. As relaxation skills develop, clients learn to differentiate Disengagement from sleep.

Lack of Relaxation Skill

A client who lacks the skills necessary to passively let go of goal-directed and analytic striving and sustain attention may simply fall asleep during relaxation training.

Lack of Sleep

A client who is tired or sleep-deprived will likely fall asleep during a relaxation session. This is a normal physiological response to a normal physiological need.

Relaxing after Eating or Consuming Alcohol

After a meal, one often feels sleepy. Blood is diverted from the brain for digestion. Consumption of alcohol, although relaxing, contributes to reductions in awareness.

Relaxing in a Position or at a Time and Place Associated with Sleep

Clients often choose to practice relaxation in a reclining position, at bedtime, in bed, or in their bedrooms. Unfortunately, such practices are likely to evoke associations of sleep and suggest that it is time to fall asleep rather than relax.

Relaxing in a Poorly Ventilated Setting

Reduced oxygen and increased carbon dioxide can contribute to feelings of drowsiness.

Consuming Medications That Can Contribute to Drowsiness

Many medications, such as common antihistamines and pain relievers, have drowsiness as a side effect. Such medications, if taken immediately before a practice session, can increase the likelihood of falling asleep.

A Wish to Avoid a Relaxation Technique, Instructor, or Setting

A client who simply does not like a technique or an instructor or a setting may respond by becoming drowsy and falling asleep.

Relaxing in a Distracting Setting

A setting may be too noisy, uncomfortable, warm, or unpleasant. A relaxation client may respond by tuning such aversive stimuli out by falling asleep.

Avoidance of N-States

Clients may become drowsy or fall asleep to avoid the threatening negative effects we considered earlier.

Avoiding External Stress Through Relaxation

At times, clients employ relaxation as a strategy for passively avoiding coping with the demands of living. For example, one may have the unpleasant duty of scheduling an income tax audit. He or she may quite innocently cope with such emotional distress by practicing a relaxation technique. However, if no action is taken or planned, relaxation may become a tool for avoiding responsibility. The relaxer may be more likely to fall asleep.

Excessive Relaxation

Clients differ in the length of practice they can tolerate. For some, 15 minutes is enough; for others, 1 hour. Clients who practice too long run the risk of falling asleep.

Misapplication of Relaxation Technique or Level

A client may practice a technique that is too advanced or simply inappropriate. Unable to effectively deploy skills related to passive attention, he or she may fall asleep.

Illness

If a client is recovering from illness or surgery, the body may need recuperative sleep.

Managing Drowsiness and Sleep in Relaxation

If sleep is temporary and occasional, it can be ignored. If a problem, the instructor may recommend:

1. Taking a nap prior to relaxation.
2. Not eating prior to relaxation.
3. If possible, not taking prescription medications before relaxation.
4. Not drinking alcoholic beverages before relaxation.
5. Practicing in a well-ventilated room.
6. Not practicing in a room associated with sleep (bedroom, lounge).
7. Not practicing at bedtime, naptime, or any other time associated with sleep.
8. Not practicing at a time when you are ordinarily most alert and awake.
9. Not practicing in a position associated with sleep (lying down, reclining).
10. Preceding preferred relaxation exercise with exercises designed to increased arousal and blood flow or the R-State Strength and Awareness (walking, singing, yoga, breathing).
11. Trying a different approach to relaxation.
12. Making a relaxation exercise shorter.
13. Making a relaxation exercise more physical.
14. Making a relaxation exercise more complex.
15. Introducing suggestions of "wakefulness" in a relaxation exercise.
16. Practicing in a group.
17. Practicing with lights on.
18. Including music or background nature sounds.

TABLE 3.1   Guidelines for Selecting a Time-Off Activity

1. Select an activity that involves a minimum of physical movement and effort. Thus, avoid jogging, sports, dancing, and similar pastimes.
2. Choose an activity that can be done alone, without outside distraction. Avoid talking over the phone, chatting with friends, playing games, engaging in sexual activity, and the like.
3. Make sure your activity is not especially goal-directed or analytic. Avoid activities that have a serious purpose, such as doing homework, practicing a musical instrument (for a class or for professional purposes), solving highly complex puzzles, doing difficult reading, planning the day's activities, or working on personal problems.
4. Pick an activity that is different from what you usually do. Try to think of something you find restful and enjoyable that you just haven't had time to do recently. Avoid activities you already do. For example, if you already spend time each day listening to pleasant music, do not choose this as your time-off activity.
5. Choose something that is indeed fun and easy. Don't make it a chore or burden. You should like doing it.
6. Take care to select an activity that will last no less than 20 minutes and no more than 30 minutes. It is important that you stick to this time period very carefully. If you are restless after 10 minutes, continue until you have finished 20 minutes (don't let your stress addiction get to you). If, after 30 minutes, you aren't finished and want to continue, stop anyway. It is important that you condition your mind and body to understand that a certain period is for time off and nothing else. Consistency and discipline are very important when teaching small children, and a stress-addicted mind and body often act like a cantankerous child. Be firm.
7. Finally, avoid the following: eating, drinking, smoking, taking drugs, sleeping.

Adapted from Smith (1989), p. 53.

TABLE 3.2   Suggested Applications of Progressive Muscle Relaxation[1]

Anger problems	Immunoincompetence
Anxiety disorders	Insomnia
Asthma	Pain, cancer
Brain injury (symptom reduction)	Pain, chronic
Chemotherapy aversion	Pain, low back
Depression	Phobias
Headache, migraine	Somatoform disorders
Headache, tension	Spasmodic dysmenorrhea
Hyperactivity	Type A behavior
Hypertension	

[1]Applications summarized from those suggested by Bernstein & Carlson, 1993; Lehrer, Carr, Sargunaraj, & Woolfolk, 1994; Lichstein, 1988; Poppen, 1998.

TABLE 3.3 Instructions for Tensing Up and Releasing Tension for Specific Muscle Groups

Smith (1989) Sequence

Hand: "Squeeze the fingers together by making a fist."

Arm: "Squeeze your lower and upper arm together, bending at the elbow. You might want to imagine you are trying to touch your shoulder with your hand."

Arm and side: "Rest your hand in your lap. Focus your attention on your arm and side and press them together, as if you were squeezing a sponge in the pit of your arm."

Back: "Focus your attention on the back muscles that are below the shoulders. Tighten up these muscles in whatever way feels best. You might arch your back (and extend your stomach and chest out) . . . or squeeze your back muscles together . . . or bend to one side and then the other . . . or even press and rub your back against the back of the chair as if you were rubbing an itch."

Shoulders: "Squeeze your shoulders in whatever way feels best . . . by shrugging them up . . . by pulling them behind you. . . . or by making a slow circling motion."

Back of neck: "Gently tilt your head back. Gently press the back of your head against your neck."

Face: "Squeeze your jaws, tongue, lip, nose, eyes, eyebrows, and forehead . . . all together. Squeeze your entire face together."

Front of neck: "Bow your head and gently press your chin down to your chest."

Stomach and chest: "Tense your stomach and chest in whatever way feels best . . . by pulling your stomach in . . . pushing it out . . . or tightening it up."

Leg: "Tense the muscles in the leg in whatever way feels best . . . by pushing your leg against the leg or back of your chair . . . or by pressing your leg tightly against the other leg."

Foot: "Curl your toes into the floor while pushing down."

Bernstein and Borkovec (1977) sequence

Hand and forearm: "Make a tight fist."

Upper arm: "Press elbow downward against the chair without involving the lower arm."

Forehead: "Raise your eyebrows as high as possible."

Upper cheeks and nose: "Squint your eyes and wrinkle your nose."

Lower face: "Clench your teeth and pull back the corners of the mouth."

Neck: "Counterpose muscles by trying to raise and lower the chin simultaneously."

Chest, shoulders, upper back: "Take a deep breath; hold it and pull shoulder blades together."

Abdomen: "Counterpose muscles by trying to push stomach out and pull it in simultaneously."

Upper leg: "Counterpose large muscle on top of the leg against the two smaller ones underneath."

Calf: "Point toes downward, turn foot in and curl toes gently."

Foot: "Point toes downward, turn foot in, and curl toes gently."

TABLE 3.4   Phrases to Be Used in PMR Patter

Tense-up Phrases
> *Tighten up the muscles.*
> *Let the tension grow.*
> *Let the tension build.*
> *Let the muscles get nice and hard.*
> *Hold the tension as if you were wringing it out.*
> *Let the feelings of tightness grow.*
> *Let the tension feel satisfying and complete.*
> *Squeeze the muscles more and more.*
> *Create a good feeling of tension.*
> *Imagine you are squeezing a rubber ball.*
> *Take care not to tense up too much.*
> *Don't tense up so it hurts.*
> *Tense up only the muscles of [NAME PART]*

Let-go Phrases
> Releasing tension
>> *Let the tension go.*
>> *Release the tension.*
>> *Let your muscles go limp.*
>> *Let the tension flow out.*
>> *Like a floppy rag doll, dropped in a chair.*
>> *Like a tight wad of paper, slowly opening up.*
>> *Let the muscles become more deeply relaxed.*
>> *Let your tension begin to unwind.*
>> *Let the muscles begin to smooth out.*
>> *Let the momentum of letting go relax you more and more thoroughly.*
>
> Reassurances of control
>> *You are in control, even when you relax.*
>> *There is nothing you have to do.*
>> *These are changes you bring about.*
>> *Notice the feelings of relaxation you can create.*
>
> Suggestions of Disengagement, Physical Relaxation, and Mental Relaxation
>> *Let yourself feel more detached.*
>> *Feelings of tension dissolve.*
>> *Let yourself forget the tensions and cares of the world.*
>> *Let yourself feel more passive.*
>> *Let yourself feel calm.*
>> *Feel relaxed.*
>> *You are at ease.*
>> *The tensions are soothed out.*
>> *As you relax, you feel more and more distant*
>
> Suggestions of cognitive tension relief
>> *Let your tensions feel soothed.*
>> *As you relax, you feel more at ease.*

TABLE 3.4   *(continued)*

Feel calm and relaxed.
Suggestions of somatic tension relief
Let yourself sink deeper and deeper into relaxation.
As you relax, your muscles become more and more heavy.
You begin to feel more and more limp.
Tension begins to melt into liquid.
As you relax, your muscles become more loose.
Phrases discriminating tension and tension relief
Compare the difference between tension and relaxation.
Notice how your muscles feel now compared with before.
Can you notice any slight feelings of tightness?
Can you notice any tension?
Compare feelings in [NAME BODY PART JUST RELAXED] with feelings in
[NAME BODY PART PREVIOUSLY RELAXED].
Phrases of increased generalization of relaxation
Let your entire body become more and more relaxed.
Let all your muscles feel more and more limp.
Let your body become increasingly relaxed.

TABLE 3.6   Suggested "Let Go" Phrases for PMR Patter

(Place this list on lap or nearby table for suggestions)

Let go.
Release the tension.
Let your muscles begin to go limp.
Let the tension begin to flow out.
Sink more and more into relaxation.
Let the muscles go limp.
There is nothing you have to do.
Let the tension begin to flow away.
Sink into relaxation.
Let the tension flow out.
Feelings of tension dissolve.
Become more limp and loose.
Let yourself relax.
Let your tension begin to unwind.
As you relax, your muscles become more and more loose.
Let yourself forget the tensions and cares of the world.
Let the tension go.
Let the rest of your body remain relaxed.
The tension melts away.
Let the muscles become more deeply relaxed.
Let your muscles go limp.
As you relax, your muscles become more loose.
You sink deeper into relaxation.
Far away from the cares of the world.
Let the muscles begin to smooth out.
Let your tension begin to unwind.
Let the tension flow out.
Let yourself sink deeper and deeper into relaxation.
Let tension dissolve.
The tension begins to flow away.
There is nothing you have to do.
And let go.
Let the muscles go completely limp.
Let tension flow away.
Let yourself relax.
Let your muscles go completely limp.
Let tension flow.
Sink more and more deeply into relaxation.
Release the tension.
Let the muscles become more and more limp.
As you relax, your muscles become more and more heavy.
You begin to feel more and more limp.
Your muscles become more and more heavy.

TABLE 3.6 *(continued)*

You sink deeper into relaxation, far away from the cares of the world.
Let the tension go.
Feelings of tightness melt and flow away.
Let yourself feel more relaxed.
Let feelings of tightness go.
Let your muscles go limp.
Release the tension.
Your back becomes more and more relaxed.
Feel the sensations of relaxation.
Let the tension flow out.
Let your tension begin to unwind.
Let the muscles begin to smooth out.
Let the muscles become more deeply relaxed.
Let the muscles go limp.
There is nothing you have to do.
Let feelings of tension dissolve.
Let the muscles become more deeply relaxed.
Let your entire body become loose and limp.
Let yourself sink deeper and deeper into relaxation.
Let yourself forget the tensions and cares of the world.
Let the tension flow away.
Your muscles feel relaxed and soothed.
As you sink far away from the cares of the world.
Feel calm and relaxed.
Let the tension smooth out.
You begin to feel more and more calm.
As you relax, you feel more at ease.
Let the tension go.
Let the tension flow out.
Let tension smooth out.
Let yourself forget the tensions and cares of the world.

TABLE 3.7   Suggested Applications of Autogenic Training

Angina pectoris
Anxiety
Asthma
Childbirth
Essential hypertension
Headaches (migraine)
Infertility
Insomnia
Myocardial infarction rehabilitation
Raynaud's disease

Applications summarized from those suggested by Linden (1993) and others.

TABLE 3.9   Suggested Applications of Breathing Exercises

Allergies
Anemia
Angina
Anxiety
Arrhythmias
Arthritis
Asthma
Bloating
Coldness of hands
Colitis
Concentration difficulties
Constipation
Depression
Diabetes
Dizziness, shakiness, trembling
Dyspnea (diaphragmatic spasm; inability to catch breath, choking sensation, feeling of
    suffocation, frequent sighing, chest heaving, lump in throat)
Epigastric pain (diaphragmatic spasm)
Fatigue
Headache (migraine)
Heart disease
Heart palpitations
Hypertension
Insomnia
Irritable bowel
Irritability
Muscle contractions (twitching; trembling; difficulty swallowing; talking; or taking
    breaths)
Musculoskeletal trauma and pain

TABLE 3.9 *(continued)*

Nausea and vomiting
Numbness and paresthesia
Obsessive compulsive disorder
Panic
Phobias
Precordial pain (intercostal muscle and diaphragmatic spasm)
Raynaud's disease
Seizures (idiopathic and organic)
Temporomandibular joint pain, bruxism

Applications summarized from those suggested by Fried, 1993; Ley, 1995.

TABLE 3.16   Script for Relaxation Voice Practice

INSTRUCTIONS: TO PRACTICE VOICES APPROPRIATE FOR DIFFERENT AP-
PROACHES TO RELAXATION, SIMPLY READ THE FOLLOWING INSTRUC-
TIONS, USING THE APPROPRIATE VOICE FOR EACH.

Progressive Muscle Relaxation (Overt)

While keeping the rest of your body loose and relaxed, shrug your shoulders *now!*
Create a nice, good squeeze. Feel it throughout your shoulder muscles.

Now let go! Let yourself go completely limp.

[PAUSE]

Let the tension begin to dissolve and flow away.

[PAUSE]

Begin to sink into a pleasant state of relaxation.

[PAUSE]

Let yourself become more and more relaxed.

[PAUSE]

Let's try that once again. Focus your attention on your shoulder muscles. And shrug
them *now!* Create a nice, good shrug. Feel the tension as it squeezes out of your shoulders.

And let go. Go completely limp.

[PAUSE]

(continued)

TABLE 3.16   *(continued)*

Let the tension begin to flow away.

[PAUSE]

Your muscles begin to feel more limp and loose as the tension flows away.

[PAUSE]

Let yourself sink deeper and deeper into relaxation.

[PAUSE]

Focus on both hands.

[PAUSE]

Tighten up both hands now.

[PAUSE]

Let the tension grow.

[PAUSE]

Feel the tension.

[PAUSE]

And go limp, resting your hands in your lap.

[PAUSE]

Let yourself go

[PAUSE]

Let the tensions begin to dissolve and flow away.

[PAUSE]

Sink deeper and deeper into pleasant relaxation.

[PAUSE]

Far away from the cares of the day.

TABLE 3.16   *(continued)*

Autogenic Exercises (Warmth/Heaviness)

Let yourself continue to sink deeper and deeper into relaxation.

Far away from the cares and concerns of the day.

There is nothing you have to do.

And quietly attend to your hands.

Let the words, "warm and heavy" float through your mind, like an echo.

[PAUSE]

Warm and heavy.

[PAUSE]

Warm and heavy.

[PAUSE]

Let these words simply float over and over, at a very slow and lazy pace.

[PAUSE]

There is nothing you have to do.

[PAUSE]

Hands and arms warm and heavy.

[PAUSE]

Like you are resting in warm sand on the beach.

[PAUSE]

Warm and heavy.

[PAUSE]

So warm and heavy as they relax more and more.

[PAUSE]

Warm and heavy, like they are sinking in warm and heavy sand.

(continued)

TABLE 3.16 *(continued)*

Yoga Stretching

Slowly, smoothly, and gently, begin to lift your right arm from your side, like the hand of a clock or the wing of a bird.

[PAUSE]

Very slowly, smoothly, and gently, as if you were balancing a feather on your hand.

[PAUSE. CONTINUE IN PACE WITH CLIENT.]

Very easily, lift your arm higher and higher.

[PAUSE. CONTINUE IN PACE WITH CLIENT.]

Take your time. Very smooth and gentle. Tracing a circle in the air.

[PAUSE, CONTINUE IN PACE WITH CLIENT.]

Lift your arm and hand over your head and reach to the sky, all the way.

[PAUSE. CONTINUE IN PACE WITH CLIENT.]

Feel the good stretch all along your arm and hand. And reach over your head, pointing to the left. Stretch every inch of your arm and hand.

[PAUSE. CONTINUE IN PACE WITH CLIENT.]

And when you are ready, gently unstretch. Very slowly, smoothly, and gently, return your arm, like the hand of a clock.

[PAUSE. CONTINUE IN PACE WITH CLIENT.]

And when you are ready, let your arm and hand hang to your side.

Breathing (Passive)

Attend to how your are breathing.

[PAUSE]

Let yourself breathe easily and naturally. Very smoothly and gently.

TABLE 3.16 *(continued)*

[PAUSE]

And now, take a full deep breath. Very smooth and even. Filling your lungs with refreshing air. And pause.

And when you are ready, slowly let the air flow out through your lips, as if you were blowing on a candle, just enough to make the flame flicker.

[PAUSE. CONTINUE IN PACE WITH CLIENT.]

And continue to breathe at a normal, relaxed pace. There is no reason to force yourself to breathe in any particular way. Just breathe easily and naturally.

[PAUSE 15 SECONDS]

And, just like before, take a slow, full breath. Very easily, fill your lungs all the way.

[PAUSE. CONTINUE IN PACE WITH CLIENT.]

When you are ready, slowly and gently exhale through your lips, as before.

[PAUSE. CONTINUE IN PACE WITH CLIENT.]

And continue to breathe naturally.

Imagery

We are now ready to explore a peaceful and relaxing story.

[PAUSE]

You can imagine any story you want, and enjoy it with all your senses.

You might imagine you have taken a long and peaceful journey. At the end of your journey you find a special cabin on a pond.

[PAUSE]

Enjoy it with all your senses.

[PAUSE]

Perhaps you can smell the clean, fresh waters and trees.

[PAUSE]

(continued)

TABLE 3.16   *(continued)*

Perhaps you hear an occasional dove singing overhead.

[PAUSE]

You may feel the refreshing touch of air and sun on your skin. Cooling. Warm. Refreshing.

[PAUSE 10 SECONDS]

The air is clear and hushed in silent expectation.

[PAUSE]

Take a few seconds to enjoy this pleasant setting. Let yourself enjoy it with all yours senses, and notice what you see, hear, feel, and smell.

[PAUSE 20 SECONDS]

And now you begin to look around.

[PAUSE]

The waters of the pond are still, like a mirror.

[PAUSE]

The cabin is warm and friendly.

[PAUSE]

In the distance a person is taking a peaceful stroll.

[PAUSE]

This place has a message of peace and wonder for you.

Perhaps it is just the good feeling of being there.

Or perhaps a special message, one just for you, appears.

TABLE 3.16 *(continued)*

Meditation

Our next exercise is called meditation. It is very simple.

Begin by calmly sitting upright in a comfortable position. Start rocking back and forth in your chair.

[PAUSE]

And now, let each movement become more and more gentle and easy. Let yourself rock effortlessly. Let your body move on its own, in its own way, at its own speed. All you have to do is simply attend.

Let each movement become more and more subtle so that someone watching would barely notice you are rocking. All you have to is quietly attend to the rocking. Every time your mind wanders, that's okay; gently return to your rocking motion.

For the next minute or so, let your rocking become barely noticeable. And quietly attend.

4

Relaxation Scripting

Over the past two decades, I have introduced relaxation to thousands of students and clients. They have taught me one very unexpected lesson. I used to think that most clients have very specific relaxation preferences and respond best to just one general strategy, whether it be progressive muscle relaxation (PMR), stretching, meditation, or another. I spent many years of research attempting to identify the PMR, yoga, or meditation "type" of person. So far I have found few patterns. All this time, my clients were teaching me something very different; virtually all preferred highly individualized mixtures of many approaches. Very few people prefer just one or two strategies alone.

This discovery has led me to develop a new approach to teaching relaxation, one based on these ideas:

1. Different approaches to relaxation have different effects and work for different people.
2. The best way to teach relaxation is not to impose one or two approaches on everyone but to introduce a variety of approaches.
3. I try to present relatively "pure" versions of each approach so that clients can discover its potential unique R-State effects unconfounded by other approaches. For example, I present PMR tense–let go cycles, minimizing breathing and imagery, so that clients can clearly note the relaxation effect of tensing up and letting go.
4. Once a client is trained in a variety of approaches, we select those that work best and construct an individualized script and tape.
5. The goal of relaxation training goes beyond the relaxation response of lowered arousal. Additional objectives are cultivating appropriate R-States and acquiring R-Beliefs that are conducive to deepening relaxation and extending its rewards to all of life.

SCRIPT WRITING

Many relaxation instructors present clients with relaxation tapes, often standardized versions available from various mental health catalogs. However, giving all clients the same tape can pose a variety of problems. Not only does such a strategy ignore client preferences, but it risks exposing clients to exercises that may have negative associations (see N-States in *ABC Relaxation Theory*). My approach is to craft for each client an individualized relaxation tape based on a mutually developed verbatim script of exercise instructions. There are several advantages to such script writing:

- You include what works for your client. (Different exercises work for different people.)
- You can select exercises for your client's relaxation goal. (Different exercises can be better for different goals.)
- Because your client is inventing his or her own relaxation exercise, he or she is more likely to take it seriously and practice it regularly. Indeed, the client may well treasure his or her script as a truly personal possession and practice it very seriously.
- Given that training is varied and changing, client interest and motivation is maintained, reducing premature quitting.
- You can include special suggestions and exercises to deepen your client's relaxation.
- Finally, your client can use relaxation as a reminder of personal philosophies conducive to living a life of peace and calm.

Even if you never intend to make individualized relaxation tapes for clients, I recommend mastering the art of script writing. Whether your preferred approach is PMR, imagery, or meditation, acquiring scripting skills will enable you to teach relaxation more effectively.

THE MECHANICS OF SCRIPT WRITING

Script writing involves making many revisions, somewhat like the process of creating a special garden. You begin with a few central pieces—for example, some rose bushes. Then you add additional flowers for color. You stand back, look at the garden, and add a little green moss here and there. After taking another look, you add some embellishments, for example, a few decorative rocks. With so many revisions and additions,

I recommend using a word processor in writing your script. An alternative method is to use 3-by-5-inch cards. When using this method, write only 1–10 words of instruction on each card ("Tense up your right hand now," "Attend to the pleasant feelings you can create"). Then, as you go through these instructions, put additional elaborations and refinements on separate cards and insert them in your expanding stack. When finished, read your entire stack of cards into a tape recorder.

When making a relaxation script and tape, first select the basic exercise components. Then return and add elaborations and deepening strategies to each basic component. Finally, fine-tune your script with a variety of refinements. Throughout the process, note your selections on the Relaxation Scripting Worksheet (Table 4.1 at end of chapter). When done, read your client's script into an audiocassette tape recorder. We will explain each step and illustrate how one imaginary person, Sue, developed her script. We conclude with some sample scripts.

The following is a summary of steps for writing a relaxation script:

1. Selection
   a. Relaxation goal
   b. Unifying idea
   c. Specific exercises
   d. Sequence and combinations
2. Elaboration
   a. Incorporation of unifying idea
   b. Imagery and meditation details
   c. Relaxation R-State words and R-Belief affirmations
   d. Coherence
3. Enhancement
   a. Deepening suggestions
   b. Deepening imagery
   c. Cascading deepening imagery
   d. Zoom imagery
   e. Deepening metaphors
   f. Deepening transitions
   g. Deepening countdowns
   h. Deepening markers
4. Refinement
   a. Anticipations of setback
   b. Relaxation reinforcements
   c. Pauses and silences
   d. Termination segment
5. Making the tape

SELECTION

The Relaxation Goal

First ask your client why he or she wants to relax. Suggest some possible goals, including managing stress, healing, combating insomnia, relaxing at the end of the day, waking up refreshed in the morning, enhancing creativity and productivity, and self-exploration and growth. Our example person, Sue, selected as her goal: "Daily relaxation for self-expression and growth."

An important part of goal selection is determining which global effects and R-States your client desires to emphasize. Several goals can be selected and can even be presented in sequence (e.g., "I first want to get away from the tensions of the day, and then feel more refreshed and aware").

To explore relaxation goals, use the Smith Relaxation Disposition/Motivations Inventory (SRDMI), the Smith Relaxation Beliefs Inventory (SRBI), and the Smith Relaxation Concerns Inventory (SCRI). All inventories are in the Appendix. For example, using these inventories, a client may identify a desire to cultivate the R-State Strength and Awareness (SRDMI), foster the R-Belief of Accepting Things that Cannot be Changed (SRBI), and manage stress and anxiety (SRCI).

Record your client's relaxation goal on your Relaxation Scripting Worksheet (*see* Table 4.1 at end of chapter).

The Unifying Idea

Traditionally, relaxation exercises are presented in a disconnected fashion, much like workout routines at a health club. In a workout one might do a few pushups, ride the exercycle, complete some situps, lift weights, and so on. Similarly, a relaxation sequence might involve a yoga standing stretch, stretching one's arms, bowing and stretching, and taking a few deep breaths. In ABC Relaxation Training, one goal is to weave exercises together so that they form a coherent whole, an integrated and meaningful sequence with a beginning, middle, and end. One tool for achieving this is the unifying idea, a statement of a sequence's justification, what it is all about. You might describe a unifying idea as an exercise's "title" that explains the gist of an exercise sequence. An exercise sequence with meaning and structure is more likely to be remembered and valued. I suggest six types of unifying ideas:

- *Exercise rationale (explanation of why it works).* Often a unifying idea is little more than the rationale of why you think it works. For example, your client may believe that relaxation is effective for reducing stress because it triggers a "relaxation response" or that it enhances creativity because it "taps the unconscious."
- *Exercise goal.* A relaxation goal can be simply the reason for practicing, for example, stress release, combating insomnia, waking up refreshed for the day, preparing for work, or even prayer or communing with nature.
- *Affirmation of an R-Belief.* Unifying ideas can be affirmations of personal relaxation philosophies; for example, "Live in the present moment," "God's will be done," "Let go of that which cannot be changed," or "Trust the powers within you."
- *Relaxation metaphor or image.* Metaphors or symbolic images of relaxation can be unifying ideas. The theme of *peaceful woods* might symbolize many types of exercises. For example, a gentle breeze might symbolize breathing exercises; trees slowly bowing in the wind, stretching exercises; and the silence of approaching evening, a meditation. Note how these images are not only peaceful in their own right but are suggestive of specific relaxation exercises. To take an example we will use later, the theme of *waves crashing on the shore* can symbolize a variety of exercises. The energy that builds and releases with each crashing wave can suggest shrugging up the shoulders and letting go as well as taking in a deep relaxing breath and exhaling tension. The dissolving of each wave into the sand can be linked with mental images suggesting "heaviness, tingling, and dissolving tension." And the quiet wind that flows across the water before the next wave can suggest relaxed breathing.
- *Relaxation story.* A unifying idea can be something of a very simple story, providing all elements are linked to relaxation exercises, change in the direction of increased relaxation, and end in deeper relaxation. For example, the theme of waves crashing on the shore is a bit of a story: a wave builds up, crashes, and dissolves into the sand, and a quiet wind blows.
- *Brief work of art.* Finally, many works of art, including poems, lyrics to songs, music, prayers, and passages from literature, can convey the essence of relaxation processes. Such artistic expressions can serve as powerful unifying themes.

It is important that your client put his or her unifying idea in their own words. Returning to our example, Sue has selected the image of sitting on the banks of a mountain stream as her unifying idea.

Select Relaxation Exercises

Next, your clients select relaxation exercises to include in their sequence in light of the selected goal(s). Selections should be highly specific. If your clients prefer yoga, ask them to list which specific stretch exercises they like. If your clients include mental imagery or fantasy, they should pick a theme that reflects their unifying idea. Be sure to write down the detailed instructions for each exercise. If you are using a word processor, each phrase (about five words) should occupy a separate line.

Sue has selected yoga stretching, breathing, imagery, and meditation as her preferred approaches. Her choices are

Back stretch (bow over and touch the ground; reach up and touch the sky)

Deep breathing

Quietly breathing out through the lips

Meditation

Sequence and Combinations

The next step is to decide on an exercise practice order consistent with the unifying idea. The default order is the sequence in which this text presents exercises—PMR, autogenic training (AT), breathing, yoga stretching, imagery, and meditation. Conversely, you might consider presenting exercises according to the R-States your client associates with each. One might begin with Disengagement and Physical Relaxation, proceed to Mental Relaxation, and conclude with Strength and Awareness, Joy, and Prayerfulness. Virtually any sequence is possible, providing it effectively conveys the client's unifying idea.

At this point it can be useful to consider one tool for sequencing and combining exercises: *crossover chaining*. A crossover exercise is one that possesses characteristics of more than one family of exercises (Smith, 1999). Such exercises can be linked, or chained, with similar exercises. For example, autogenic warmth/heaviness suggestions have both a somatic (the sensation of warmth and heaviness) and internal visual (imagining warm water on the hand) component. As such, warmth/heaviness suggestions can flow naturally from more purely somatic techniques, such as PMR, to sense imagery. Similarly, many active stretching exercises, such as bowing and exhaling and reaching up while inhaling, fall in the families of movement/posture and breathing. Because of this, stretching and breathing exercises can often be chained. Below are a number of possible crossover chains.

Autogenic warmth/heaviness→imagery for autogenic warmth/heaviness→sense imagery→insight imagery→meditation imagery

Yoga stretching→stretching + breathing→breathing→breath meditation

Overt PMR→covert PMR phased with breathing→breathing

Deep breathing→restful singing or chanting paced with breathing→simple repetitive prayer→mantra meditation involving one or two words from preceding prayer

We are now ready to examine excerpts from Sue's script. (See Table 4.2.) Detailed instructions for yoga and breathing are presented; those for imagery have been left for later.

ELABORATION

Incorporation of Unifying Idea

Each exercise your client has selected should be linked with the unifying idea. Explain to your client the importance of this step, something like stringing beads on a chain. For example, in the following segment the

TABLE 4.2   Sue's Script: Exercise Selection and Sequence

Yoga Stretch

Sit up slowly, smoothly, and gently. Reach and stretch higher and higher into the sky, as if you were touching the clouds. Reach all the way. And then pause. Then, slowly, smoothly, and gently return to an upright, seated position.

Breathing

Take in a deep breath, filling your lungs completely.

Gently exhale.

Let the air flow out of your lips with every breath.

Imagery: Sitting on the Banks of a Mountain Stream. To Be Aadded Later.

Meditation

unifying idea is "breathing out tension and settling into calm." Notice how this idea is woven into each exercise:

Take in a deep breath. Slowly bow over, let go, and exhale.
Let tension begin to melt and flow out with your breath.
Now we become more calm. While sitting upright, breathe in deeply and slowly and exhale. As you begin to settle into calm, let more and more tension dissolve and float away.
Now, let yourself become even more calm. Let your breathing be effortless and unforced. Simply attend to each incoming and outgoing breath. Let yourself settle into a deeper and deeper state of relaxation as any remaining tension begins to flow away.

As we noted earlier, a unifying idea can also be expressed in a simple story—for example, "a leaf floating down the river," "a bubble rising to the surface of the pond," or "the sun dissolving a block of ice into a puddle of water." Here is an example in which such story changes are woven into a sequence of exercises:

Tense and let go. Imagine a bubble released from the floor of a pond.
Quietly attend to your breathing. Let tension flow with every outgoing breath. As breath flows, the bubble slowly rises.
In your mind's eye simply attend to the bubble as it reaches the surface. It touches the air and bursts, releasing its tension. Let go of remaining feelings of tension.

Here are some more examples of how to weave a unifying idea into an exercise sequence.

Unifying Idea: The Relaxation Goal of Preparing for Sleep

Tense up your shoulders. Let go. Release some of the tension that keeps you from sinking deeper into a pleasant drowsy state.
Take in a deep breath. Let the air soothe you and calm your tensions. Let the air out and sink into sleepiness
Quietly breathe in and out. With each outgoing breath, let yourself become more quiet and drowsy.
Imagine a quiet forest, a dreamlike image as you sink into drowsiness.

Unifying Idea: A Personal Relaxation Philosophy: "Let Go of Needless Control."

Tense up your shoulders. Notice how this is like trying to control your life. Now relax and let go. Let go of the needless tension you have created.

Take in a deep breath. Hold it in, as you hold in needless tension through the day. Then relax and breathe out, letting go of needless tension.

Imagine in your mind a flowing stream. The stream is peaceful, flowing through life without needless control.

Unifying Idea: The Image of a Ball of String Unwinding

Tense up your shoulder muscles. Imagine tension as a tight ball of string. Then relax and let go. Imagine the ball of string slowly unwinding.

Take in a deep breath. Hold it in. Then relax and breathe out. The ball of string unwinds even more.

Unifying Idea: A Palm Tree Bowing in the Wind

Imagine you are a palm tree bowing gently in the wind.
You are on a very peaceful island, far away from any cares and concerns.
The wind blows, and subsides.
As the wind begins to blow, tense, let go, and gently stretch.
Stretch farther and farther, feeling a full and comfortable stretch.
And as the wind subsides, gently unstretch, releasing your tension.
As you become more relaxed, attend to the flow of breath.
Imagine a gentle breeze flowing by as you gently breathe in and out.

Unifying Idea: A Modified Fragment of the "Serenity Prayer": "Help Me to Tend to That Which Truly Matters, to Let Go of That Which Does Not Matter, and to Know the Difference."

Calmly meditate to the word *peace*. Let it float through your mind.
"Peace . . . Peace." Tend to that which truly matters.
Gently tense up. Let go, and release the tension.
Let go of that which does not matter.
It is peace that truly matters.
Breathe gently and easily.
With each breath, think: "Peace . . . peace . . . peace."

Here again is Sue's script (Table 4.3). Note how her unifying idea, the image of sitting on the bank of a mountain stream, is repeated in each exercise.

Imagery and Meditation Details

If your client has selected imagery, visualization, fantasy, or meditation to be a part of his or her script, now is the time to elaborate and add

TABLE 4.3 Sue's Script: Unifying Idea (New Additions in Italics)

Yoga Stretch

Imagine you are sitting on the banks of a mountain stream. You bow over, gently touching the water. Let tension dissolve into the water.

Sit up slowly, smoothly, and gently. Reach and stretch higher and higher into the sky, as if you were touching the clouds. Reach all the way. And then pause. Then, slowly, smoothly, and gently return to an upright, seated position.

Breathing

Take in a deep breath, filling your lungs completely.

Gently exhale.

Let the air flow out of your lips with every breath.

The only sound you hear is the quiet flow of breath and a quiet mountain stream.

Imagery: Sitting on the Banks of a Mountain Stream

Meditation

---

details. The same is true if your client wants a meditation. Select the meditation focus. Once again, tie the details in with the unifying idea. We will now take a look just at Sue's imagery and meditation exercises (Table 4.4).

Relaxation R-State Words and R-Belief Affirmations

You can enhance and "spice up" your client's exercise sequence with words your client picks from the extended relaxation word list (Table 4.5 at end of chapter). Select words consistent with the desired R-States. Consider beginning with words suggesting Disengagement and Physical Relaxation and ending with words suggesting Strength and Awareness, Joy, Love and Thankfulness, and Prayerfulness.

You can also add phrases that affirm your client's R-Beliefs (below). These should be introduced no more than once every 10 sentences. Here are some I have identified:

**TABLE 4.4 Sue's Script: Imagery and
Meditation Elaborations (New Additions in Italics)**

Imagery: Sitting on the Banks of a Mountain Stream

*Now, quietly attend only to the image of sitting on the banks of
a cool, refreshing mountain stream.*

Your feet gently swing in the cool, refreshing water.

*Tension flows down each leg, into your toes, and is dissolved
and carried away by the water.*

*You can see the clear, sparkling water, smell its clean spray,
and feel the warm sun on your skin.*

*Attend with all of your senses to this beautiful, relaxing
moment.*

Meditation

Quietly attend to the coming and going of the present moment.

Belief 1: View the world with optimism.
   I can be optimistic about my current hassles.
   It is important to be optimistic.
Belief 2: Accept things the way they are.
   I can accept things as they are.
   There's no need to try to change what can't be changed.
Belief 3: Be honest with yourself and others.
   I can accept my thoughts and feelings.
   I can be honest and open with my feelings.
Belief 4: Know when to let go and take it easy.
   Sometimes it is important to simply take it easy.
   It is important to know when to stop trying, let go, and relax.
Belief 5: Relate to others with love and compassion.
   *The love I give and receive is a source of peace and comfort
      to me.*
   *It is important to treat people with compassion and under-
      standing.*
Belief 6: Trust the healing wisdom of the body.
   I trust the body's wisdom and healing powers.
   There are sources of strength and healing deep within me.

Belief 7: Trust God's love and guidance.
   God guides, loves, and comforts me.
   I put myself in God's hands.
Belief 8: Put your concerns in deeper perspective.
   Life has a purpose greater than my personal wants and desires.
   There's more to life than my personal concerns and worries.

If a poem, passage of literature, prayer, or lyrics of a song express what relaxation means to your client, by all means try to weave it into the script.

We can now return to Sue. She has selected the phrases "become more and more still," "sink more and more deeply into a pleasant state of relaxation," "your mind becomes peacefully centered," and "time is like a river; each crises passes and is forgotten." Note how these, plus such phrases as "let the tension . . . let tension dissolve," enhance relaxation (*see* Table 4.6).

Coherence

An exercise sequence that is just a random chain of calisthenics is uninteresting and easily forgotten. A number of strategies can enhance the coherence of a sequence, the degree to which separate parts fit together.

If your client's relaxation sequence includes several general approaches (e.g., yoga and breathing and meditation), elements of one approach can be integrated into others. For example, breathing exercises can be separately featured in a relaxation sequence or woven into tense–let go or yoga stretching:

Take a deep breath as you tighten up the muscles.
Hold the muscles tighter and tighter.
As you let go, gently exhale.
Slowly, smoothly, and gently stretch.
Stretch farther and farther.
Gently take in a deep breath as you stretch completely.
And very slowly, smoothly, and gently release the stretch while exhaling.

Similarly, if your client likes imagery and fantasy, specific images can be integrated into other physical exercises in order to weave them together:

TABLE 4.6 Sue's Script: Phrases Suggesting the Deepening of Relaxation (New Additions in Italics)

Yoga Stretch

Imagine you are sitting on the banks of a mountain stream. You bow over, gently touching the water. Let tension dissolve into the water.

Sit up slowly, smoothly, and gently. Reach and stretch higher and higher into the sky, as if you were touching the clouds. Reach all the way. And then pause. Then, slowly, smoothly, and gently return to an upright, seated position.

Sink more and more deeply into a pleasant state of relaxation.

Breathing

Take in a deep breath, filling your lungs completely.

Gently exhale.

Become more and more still.

Let the air flow out of your lips with every breath.

The only sound you hear is the quiet flow of breath and a quiet mountain stream.

Imagery: Sitting on the Banks of a Mountain Stream

Now, quietly attend only to the image of sitting on the banks of a cool, refreshing mountain stream.

Become more and more still.

Your feet gently swing in the cool, refreshing water.

Tension flows down each leg, into your toes, and is dissolved and carried away by the water.

You can see the clear, sparkling water, smell its clean spray, and feel the warm sun on your skin.

Your mind becomes peacefully centered.

Time is like a river, each crisis passes and is forgotten.

Attend with all of your senses to this beautiful, relaxing moment.

Meditation

Quietly attend to the coming and going of the present moment.

As you let go of your tension, imagine a tight ball of string slowly unwinding. Bit by bit each string relaxes as you let go of tension more and more completely. Gently and easily, the entire wad becomes more and more loose.

As you stretch, imagine you are a tree. Your arms are the branches gracefully bending in the wind. With every breeze, you bend and release your tensions.

You are by the seashore. As each wave approaches the shore, you take a deep breath. As the wave splashes against the shore, you gently exhale and release your tensions.

Returning to Sue, we can see that she has introduced repeated instructions for "exhaling through lips" to help add unity to her sequence.

TABLE 4.7   Sue's Script: Coherence (New Additions in Italics)

Yoga Stretch

Imagine you are sitting on the banks of a mountain stream. You bow over, gently touching the water. Let tension dissolve into the water.

Sit up slowly, smoothly, and gently. Reach and stretch higher and higher into the sky, as if you were touching the clouds. Reach all the way. And then pause. Then, slowly, smoothly, and gently return to an upright, seated position.

Sink more and more deeply into a pleasant state of relaxation.

Quietly open your lips, and let tension flow with every breath.

Let the flow of breath be as gentle as the flow of a quiet mountain stream.

Breathing

Take in a deep breath, filling your lungs completely.

Gently exhale.

Become more and more still.

Let the air flow out of your lips with every breath.

The only sound you hear is the quiet flow of breath and a quiet mountain stream.

(continued)

TABLE 4.7 *(continued)*

Let your flow of breath be as gentle as a mountain stream.

Imagery: Sitting on the Banks of a Mountain Stream

Now, quietly attend only to the image of sitting on the banks of a cool, refreshing mountain stream.

Become more and more still.

Your feet gently swing in the cool, refreshing water.

Tension flows down each leg, into your toes, and is dissolved and carried away by the water.

Quietly open your lips and let tension flow with every breath.

The flow of breath is as gentle as a mountain stream.

With every outgoing breath, let go of your worries over past and future.

You can see the clear, sparkling water, smell its clean spray, and feel the warm sun on your skin.

Your mind becomes peacefully centered.

Time is like a river; each crisis passes and is forgotten.

Attend with all of your senses to this beautiful, relaxing moment.

Meditation

Quietly attend to the coming and going of the present moment.

ENHANCEMENT

A number of deepening strategies can enhance sustained passive simple focus.

Deepening Suggestions

Perhaps the simplest deepening strategy is to incorporate R-State words as suggestions of movement and change. For example, the simple suggestion

"You are relaxed" can be made into a deepening suggestion: "You are becoming more and more relaxed." Similarly one can say, "You are becoming more distant," "more strengthened and aware," "more joyful," and so on.

Deepening Imagery

Deepening imagery reflects our attentional definition of relaxation. Such imagery begins by being relatively active, complex, and discursive (moving to and fro) and then becomes increasingly passive, simple, and focused. We can see this in the following example:

You are relaxing on a beach. As you sit up and look around, you notice the blue water and sky. The sun is directly overhead, its warm rays dissolving tension in your body. You can feel the wind and hear the soothing waves splash against the shore. As you become more relaxed, you recline on the beach. The wind dies down to a gentle breeze. Your attention narrows to the sky above and the peaceful clouds floating by. There is nothing you have to think about or do. The air is now completely still The sea is silent. Simply attend to the clouds and nothing else.

NOTE ACTIVITIES: "SITTING UP, LOOKING, NOTICING." COMPLEX IMAGES INVOLVING MOVEMENT AND ACTIVITY ("BLOWING WIND," "SPLASHING WAVES"

A MORE PASSIVE POSTURE WIND BECOMES MORE PASSIVE.

NOTE INCREASE IN SIMPLE FOCUS

VERY PASSIVE. AIR AND SEA ARE STILL. VERY SIMPLE FOCUS.

Cascading Deepening Imagery

A cascading deepening image is a sequence of linked deepening images. Each image begins as active, complex, and discursive and ends as passive, simple, and focused. However, the ending of one image serves as the beginning of another image and, in the context of what follows, is relatively active, complex, and discursive. Notice how the two images below, one of a rainstorm and one of a waterfall, have been linked. The beginning rainstorm is active, complex, and discursive. Much is going on in the image: thunder, lightning, and a rapidly flowing stream. This image then becomes more passive, simple, and focused as the storm subsides and the stream settles to a ripple. The end of this image is a quiet and simple waterfall. The waterfall then becomes the beginning of another deepening image. It now is relatively active, complex, and discursive. We see water splashing on many rocks and hear the sounds of water flowing and bubbling. We follow the flow of water to a passive, simple, and quiet pond. And our attention is again focused.

You are safe and sound in a forest cabin. It is raining outside. You hear the wind blowing hard and the thunder in the distance. A torrent of rain pours against the roof and windows. But you are safe inside, beside a warm fireplace. The outside turbulence seems a distant concern.

Gradually, the rain begins to subside, the wind grows quiet, and the thunderclouds float away. Looking outside, you can see the weather clearing. The air is calm and still. And in the distance, you can see a waterfall, the water quietly rushing over the rocks.

As you settle into quiet relaxation, your attention dwells on the waterfall. You notice it splashing over rocks, catching an occasional twig and leaf as it flows into hundreds of tiny eddies. You notice the soothing sound of bubbling water, the rushing of water against the rocks and shore and, in the distance, the waterfall itself. As you become more relaxed and calm, your attention centers on a small swirl of water in the pond below the water. You notice the water slowly circling, again and again. You attend to this simple motion.

Zoom Imagery

Zoom imagery is a variant of deepening imagery. Here the inclusiveness of an image broadens or narrows, resulting in a reduction of activity, complexity, and discursiveness and an increase in passive simple focus. With *open focus zoom imagery*, one's stance regarding a focal stimulus recedes, including more and more surrounding stimuli. As a result, the target stimulus is seen with increased perspective and detachment. Details, which once may have contributed to activity, complexity, and discursiveness, become less prominent. Here is an example:

Attend to a small flower in the field. Notice the detail in its red petals, drops of dew, and a buzzing insect busily gathering pollen. The flower shimmers as the breeze flows by. This is a small world alive with activity and energy. Slowly, we move above the flower and notice it is in a cluster of flowers, each swaying in the wind. We no longer notice the occasional bee as we move further away. As we continue to step back, the flowers merge into a colorful garden, filled with soft pastel colors. Seen as a whole, the garden is still, at peace, a rainbow of stillness.

Another image, almost a cliche in this day of space exploration, dramatically illustrates the effect of open focus zoom imagery.

You are resting on the grass in a busy park. Children play. Dogs and cats run about. A small band plays in the distance. Much is going on. Imagine yourself slowly and safely rising into the air. At first only a few feet; you see the ground directly below. Then a few more feet, and you can see the tops of bushes, then of trees. As you rise further and further, you see more of the park below, then the lake near the park. Soon you see an entire landscape vista begin to unfold below— rivers, lakes, cities. Eventually, you are far in space, looking at the serene blue orb of earth. Everything is so peaceful and quiet when seen in this perspective.

Centered focus zoom imagery moves in the opposite direction. One moves closer to the object of attention, excluding stimuli that are extraneous active, complex, and discursive. Here's an example:

Imagine you are seated next to a waterfall and a pond. You notice the spray of water as it cascades across the rocks and splashes onto surrounding trees and into the water. You notice the foaming water below, as floating leaves and twigs rise and fall. Your attention is drawn to one shiny rock, the size of closed hand. The rock is smooth from ages of flowing water. As your attention focuses on the rock, slowly you forget the spray of water around, the bubbling pond, and all the surrounding sounds. The shiny rock, in its peaceful simplicity, becomes the focus of your attention.

Deepening Metaphors

The use of metaphors can enhance relaxation by symbolizing both concrete exercise procedures and R-Beliefs. A swaying tree can signify a yoga stretch or the philosophical statement "Flow with the here and now."

Crashing ocean waves can signify the exhalation of breath or a commitment to "let go of that which cannot be changed." Such metaphors are, in a sense, more abstract than exercises and more concrete than R-Beliefs. Because they exist at an intermediate level of abstraction, they can be used to foster transitions from concrete exercises to affirmations of R-Beliefs, as illustrated here:

Stretch and unstretch your arms.
Stretch and unstretch your legs.
With each stretch, you are like a tree swaying in the wind.
Stretch, unstretch, and sway in the wind.
A tree sways in the wind, firmly rooted in the earth, yet flowing with the moment.
Remember how you, firmly supported by the ground of life, can flow with the moment.

Deepening Transitions

If more than one exercise is selected for a script, deepening transitions can be introduced between each. Such transitions reinforce the thought that exercises are not an arbitrary assortment but lead into further relaxation. A transition phrase can be as simple as this: "We have now completed one exercise and will move on to an exercise that is even more passive and calm."

Such transitions can incorporate any R-State, for example, "As we proceed, you feel more Strengthened and Aware." One might also cultivate a more general expectation of change: "Something wonderful is about to happen," "You will discover something very interesting," "You will discover a message of peace of serenity."

Deepening Countdowns

Another way to deepen relaxation is to introduce a relaxation countdown. Start with any number, usually 5 or 10, and slowly count back to 1. Each count is associated with increased level of an R-State. Introduce the countdown with an explanation of the countdown, for example: "We will now count from five to one. With each number, let yourself become more relaxed."

Then slowly proceed with the count, introducing a transitional suggestion between each number:

Five . . .
Let yourself become more relaxed.
Four . . .
Let feelings of tension flow away.
Three . . .
Notice how you feel as you become increasingly calm.
Two . . .
Your entire body becomes calm and relaxed.
And one . . .
Enjoy the feelings of relaxation you have created.

Countdowns can be woven into any approach to relaxation. For example, PMR "let-go patter" can include a countdown. In stretching and breathing sequences, countdowns can be incorporated into unstretching and exhaling. Imagery provides the richest opportunity for the countdown strategy. Here the actual content of an image can change or reflect increased tension relief, disengagement, or engagement, as illustrated below.

"In this exercise you will imagine yourself beginning to float into the air. I will count from one to five. With each count you will feel more relaxed, calm, and peaceful."

Five . . .
You begin to float. As you let go of your tensions, you become lighter and lighter.
Four . . .
Your mind centers on the peaceful sensations of floating and relaxation.
Three . . .
You float higher and higher. The houses and trees below become smaller and smaller. Your everyday pressures and concerns seem so distant.
Two . . .
As you approach the peaceful soft clouds, your mind feels more and more free, more and more open to the possibilities of relaxation.
One . . .
You float into the clouds, completely without effort and concern. You feel free and peaceful.

Deepening Markers

Deepening markers are very similar to countdowns. A relaxation word or exercise element can acquire meaning from the context of surrounding exercises. For example, the phrase "let go" has a concrete meaning in PMR ("let go of the tension in your hands"). The same phrase can be an affirmation of an R-Belief in a different context ("Remember that you can trust in God. It is okay to *let go* of your personal hassles and concerns"). A deepening marker is a relaxation word or exercise strategically repeated through an exercise sequence. Each time the marker appears, it is in a different context of surrounding exercises and acquires new, deeper meaning. Such repetition reinforces the suggestion of movement in relaxation. In the following example, the simple act of exhalation is a marker.

> Let yourself become more relaxed with every breath.
> Let tension begin to dissolve and flow away.
> You sink deeper and deeper into relaxation.
> Take a deep breath, and slowly exhale.
> Let muscle tension flow away as you exhale.
> You sink into deeper relaxation.
> Far away from the cares of the world.
> There is nothing to do or think about.
> Let your worries flow away with every breath you exhale.
> Your cares are as light as the breath you breathe.
> Sink even more deeply into relaxation.
> Far from your worries.
> Into a private world of inner calm.
> Let yourself inhale and exhale freely and easily, without effort.
> Live one day at a time.
> Do not try to change that which cannot be changed.
> The flow of breath is free and easy, like the coming and going of each moment.

The following example incorporates PMR, breathing, imagery, and mantra meditation. The marking phrase "let it be" is introduced in each part of the sequence; however, it acquires subtle new meanings depending on its context. Here are excerpts of the sequence:

PMR

> Tighten up and shrug the shoulder muscles.
> Let the tension grow.
> Create a nice complete squeeze in your shoulders.
> And let go.
> *Let it be.*

Let the tension begin to flow from your shoulders.
Let your shoulders become more and more relaxed and limp.
There is nothing you have to do but let it be.

Breathing

Slowly take in a complete breath.
Fill your lungs with air.
Pause.
And relax, letting the air flow.
Easily exhale.
And now let yourself breathe at a natural pace, without trying to make yourself breathe in any particular way.
Simply let yourself breathe. *Let it be.* Let the air flow in and out on its own.

Insight Imagery

And we complete our journey through the forest and discover a flat and shiny rock on the ground.
Your first urge is to lift the rock and see what secrets are underneath.
You *let it be*, and simply attend to the rock's shimmering surface.
The rock has a message of peace for you, which will appear if you simply and calmly attend. You *let it be*, and attend to what the rock has to say.

Meditation

Calmly, the words "*let it be*" slowly float through your mind like an echo.
There is nothing you have to do. Quietly attend to the words, as they go over and over in your mind. Whenever your mind wanders, that's okay. Simply return to attending to the words "*let it be.*"

REFINEMENT

Anticipations of Setback

You are now about finished with your client's script. In relaxation, setbacks are common: attention wanders, expected relaxation effects do not occur, unexpected experiences are encountered, one forgets to practice, negative thoughts interfere with relaxation, coping failures in everyday life increase tension, and so on. It is useful to expect such setbacks and deal with them through special phrases introduced in your script (e.g., "Distractions are normal, and can indicate that relaxation is uncovering hidden stresses; relaxation is like any other skill, it takes time to work; sometimes deeper levels of relaxation can create unexpected feelings and sensations"). Here are some more examples:

> Whenever you notice you are thinking about something unrelated to relaxation, picture yourself letting go of this thought as if it were a butterfly you are holding and releasing.
> Give each distracting thought to your relaxation as if you were giving it a gift.
> Say to yourself, "What an interesting distraction. OK, back to my relaxation."
> Say to the distraction "thank you" and return to your exercise.
> Imagine dropping each distraction into a deep space as though you were dropping pebbles into a pond.
> Let distracting thoughts and pictures stay in your mind if they want to. But they stay in the background while you return to your exercise.
> Imagine each distraction to be a form of stress release that enables you to relax better.

Relaxation Reinforcements

One way of deepening and strengthening relaxation is to introduce a few words of encouragement and support and highlight pleasurable, rewarding aspects of relaxation. Such reinforcements can be presented as direct statements ("Very good") or as phrases combined with other instructions ("It is good to let go of the cares of the day"). Such reinforcing phrases include the following:

> There is no need to push yourself, you are doing fine.
> Move at a pace that feels comfortable to you.
> Notice the pleasant feelings you have created.
> It is OK to let yourself sink deeper into relaxation.
> When you let go and attend to relaxation, you are doing well.

Take care not to introduce reinforcements for thoughts your client may not have. For example, the reinforcement, "It is good that you are completely relaxed" may for some clients create needless worry and tension if they are not in fact completely relaxed. It is better to reinforce relaxation attempts ("It is good to begin to put aside the cares of the day") as well as the general direction (and not the end point) of relaxation ("It is good to become more focused").

It is important to withhold reinforcements from thoughts not conducive to relaxation. For example, it is OK to experience distraction during a session. However, pursuing distractions for any length of time serves to reinforce the initial decision to pursue. Also, by reacting to distraction with a considerable degree of disturbance and upset, one appraises the distraction as major and important. It is better to treat distractions as passing and insignificant.

Sue's reinforcements are tied in with her affirmation of an R-Belief: "In this silent moment you realize that all things come and go. It is good. You are doing fine. It is a time of deep inner peace and joy."

Pauses and Silences

A relaxation sequence should include frequent pauses and periods of silence. It is at moments when nothing is being said or done that the effects of an exercise can begin to take hold. There are also times during an exercise when your client might want to be left in silence, for example, during meditation. Finally, beginning script writers tend to be too stingy with pauses; it is better to write in too many than too few.

Termination Segment

A relaxation sequence should not end abruptly. To do so might result in disruptive continuation of Disengagement into wakefulness. Gently state that the relaxation sequence is now over. Gradually return to the outside world and end with a good stretch or deep breath. A termination segment can include a suggestion that the pleasant feelings of relaxation will carry over to the rest of the day.

We are now ready to take a look at Sue's script, including her anticipation of setback, reinforcing segment, pauses, and termination segment (*see* Table 4.8).

TABLE 4.8   Sue's Final Script (New Additions in Italics)

Yoga Stretch

Imagine you are sitting on the banks of a mountain stream. You bow over, gently touching the water. Let tension dissolve into the water.

PAUSE

Sit up slowly, smoothly, and gently. Reach and stretch higher and higher into the sky, as if you were touching the clouds. Reach all the way. And then pause. Then, slowly, smoothly, and gently return to an upright, seated position.

PAUSE

Sink more and more deeply into a pleasant state of relaxation.

PAUSE

Quietly open your lips, and let tension flow with every breath.

PAUSE

Let the flow of breath be as gentle as the flow of a quiet mountain stream.

PAUSE 10 SECONDS.

Breathing

Take in a deep breath, filling your lungs completely.

Gently exhale.

PAUSE

Become more and more still.

PAUSE

Let the air flow out of your lips with every breath.

PAUSE

The only sound you hear is the quiet flow of breath and a quiet mountain stream.

PAUSE

Let your flow of breath be as gentle as a mountain stream.

PAUSE 15 SECONDS.

TABLE 4.8 *(continued)*

Imagery: Sitting on the Banks of a Mountain Stream

Now, quietly attend only to the image of sitting on the banks of a cool, refreshing mountain stream.

PAUSE

Become more and more still.

PAUSE

Your feet gently swing in the cool, refreshing water.

PAUSE

Tension flows down each leg, into your toes, and is dissolved and carried away by the water.

PAUSE

Quietly open your lips and let tension flow with every breath.

PAUSE

The flow of breath is as gentle as a mountain stream.

PAUSE

With every outgoing breath, let go of your worries over past and future.

PAUSE

You can see the clear, sparkling water, smell its clean spray, and feel the warm sun on your skin.

PAUSE

Your mind becomes peacefully centered.

PAUSE

Time is like a river; each crisis passes and is forgotten.

Let yourself relax at your own pace; if your mind wanders from time to time, that's fine.

PAUSE

Attend with all of your senses to this beautiful, relaxing moment.

PAUSE 1 MINUTE.

(continued)

TABLE 4.8 *(continued)*

Meditation

Quietly attend to the coming and going of the present moment.

If you are distracted, that's OK; simply return to your relaxation.

PAUSE 5 MINUTES.

In this silent moment you realize that all things come and go. It is good. You are doing fine. It is time of deep inner peace and joy.

PAUSE 1 MINUTE.

Take in a deep breath.

And exhale.

Gently let go of what you are attending to.

With every outgoing breath, let your eyes slowly open to the outside world.

This concludes the relaxation script.

EVALUATING YOUR SCRIPT

Once you have written your client's script, it is useful to check for possible problems. Are the instructions concrete and specific? Include every detail and leave very little to the imagination. Remember that you do not want your client to be concerned with filling in missing details or figuring out what ambiguous instructions mean. So instead of saying "Do some yoga stretching with your arm," say "Slowly, smoothly, and gently stretch and reach with your right arm." This instruction is far too vague: "Imagine a cool pond and relax." This one is better: "Picture yourself next to a clear, cool pond. There is barely a ripple. The water is blue. The sky is clear without a cloud. You can feel a calm wind."

Examine your client's script for statements that might be questioned. Avoid phrases like "You will immediately recover from your cold," "You will find the answer to your problem."

Frankly, your client may not immediately recover from a cold, find an answer to a problem, or become more relaxed than ever. So avoid making promises you might not be able to keep.

Be attentive to the possibility that your client may have difficulties with absolutistic statements, such as "Become completely relaxed," "Sink more deeply into relaxation than you have ever sunk before," "You will experience the deepest peace you can imagine at this moment." For some clients, such statements can enhance and deepen relaxation. However, others find absolutistic statements worrisome ("What if I'm very relaxed but not 'completely' relaxed?" "Just how far is 'sinking deeper than I have ever sunk before'?" If problems arise, change absolutistic statements into relative statements that cannot be questioned: "Become *more* relaxed," "Sink *deeper*," "Experience *deep peace*."

Avoid abruptly introducing exercise elements or images without a previously established context. For example, in the following exercise, the image of a candle flame seems to be arbitrarily introduced:

Your hands feel warm and heavy, warm and heavy.
With every outgoing breath, feel warm and heavy, warm and heavy.
Let your breathing be slow and easy, as your hands become warm and heavy.
Your breathing is slow and easy and relaxed.
Attend to the candle flame in front of you.

Here the image of a candle flame is given a context.

You are seated by a candle, relaxing in the glowing light it provides.
On your hands, you can feel its warmth.
Your hands feel warm and heavy, warm and heavy.
Let your breathing be slow and easy, so gentle you barely cause the
candle flame to flicker.
And your hands feel warm and heavy.
Your breathing is slow and easy and relaxed.
As you attend to the flame in front of you, one that burns and flickers
freely and effortlessly.

Check if your client is comfortable with the quantity and quality of
verbal description you have included. Some clients want to be left alone
in a relaxation exercise, with relatively little verbal patter. Others prefer
to have their exercise filled with patter. Similarly, some clients are uncomfortable with too much visual and poetic imagery; others prefer it.

HOW TO MAKE AN AUDIOCASSETTE TAPE

You do not have to be an accomplished actor to record an relaxation
audiocassette tape. Simply read your script instructions into a tape recorder.
However, a few guidelines can help you do your best.

- Speak slowly. Most beginning relaxation tape makers (and a few
  famous professionals who should know better) speak too quickly.
- Speak softly in a monotone. You are not giving a lecture or talking
  across the hall to someone with a hearing impairment.
- When comfortable, moderate your voice to the type of relaxation
  you are presenting. Use your "PMR or AT voice," "yoga voice,"
  "breathing voice," "imagery voice," and "meditation voice."
- When presenting PMR instructions, keep talking.
- Most beginners are stingy with pauses and silences. Pauses and
  silences are essential to relaxation and provide the client with time
  to complete instructions and enjoy their effects. If you are going to
  make a mistake, make your pauses and silences too long rather than
  too short. Few things are more annoying than a rushed relaxation
  script.

EXTENDED EXAMPLES

Exercises   (See if you can note the
                                   scripting principles deployed)

Muscle Relaxation

Goal: General stress management
Unifying idea: Detecting, releasing
muscle tension.

In this exercise we are going to quietly look for and release sources of muscle tension. We will do this several ways, first by actively squeezing and letting go, then letting go as we exhale and release our breath, and finally by engaging in a special type of mental imagery. Note that we will shift from active to passive, not only in each exercise but in the entire sequence.

Take in a deep breath, and tighten up your hand muscles *now*.

Hold the tension.

Notice how tension feels.

And *let go*, gently letting out all the air. That's good.

[PAUSE]

Let the tension begin to flow out of your fingers.

[PAUSE]

Study the difference between sensations of tension and relaxation.

[PAUSE]

As your fingers become more relaxed, think the words "fingers warm and heavy, fingers warm and heavy."

[PAUSE]

Attend to the sensations of relaxation as you sink into relaxation.
[REPEAT TWICE FOR EVERY MAJOR MUSCLE GROUP.]
And now we move to exercises that are more gentle.

Slowly take in a deep breath.
[PAUSE]
Notice any feelings of tension you may have.
[PAUSE]
And gently *let go*.
[PAUSE]
Let tightness flow out as you exhale.
[PAUSE]
Let the flow of air bring warmth and heaviness to your fingers, hands, arms, and feet as you sink deeper into relaxation.
[PAUSE]
Compare the subtle sensations of tension and relaxation.
[PAUSE]
It's OK to let yourself have feelings of warmth, tingling, or heaviness.
As we continue, our exercises become more and more passive and quiet.
Let our breathing continue easily and unforced.
[PAUSE]
Quietly attend to your hands and fingers.
[PAUSE]
Imagine a warm stream of air gently caressing your hands and fingers.
[PAUSE]

The flow of air dissolves your tensions and carries them away.
[PAUSE]

Very slowly and gently, the flow of air starts at your wrist and smoothes out remaining tension all the way to the fingertips. Picture tension as tiny wrinkles that are easily smoothed into relaxation.
[PAUSE 15 SECONDS.]

Let yourself sink more and more deeply into a pleasant state of relaxation. Your mind focuses more and more on the calm you have created.
[REPEAT FOR ARMS, BACK, SHOULDERS, NECK, FACE, LEGS, AND FEET.]

Let yourself relax.

Quietly attend to the feelings you have created.
[PAUSE]

Gently open your eyes.

Stretch your neck as you look around.

This completes our relaxation sequence.

A Yoga Stretching Meditation

Goal: Recovering from a hectic day
Unifying idea: A palm tree bowing in the wind

Imagine you are a palm tree standing by the ocean beach. As the wind blows, big waves crash against the shore. Each wave releases its tension as the water runs up and dissolves into the sand. The warm sun shines overhead, a source of life and energy for all the world.

[PAUSE]

A long, slow gust of wind sighs through the leaves.

[PAUSE]

Slowly, smoothly, and gently bow over and stretch completely.

[PAUSE]

Feel the stretch completely, all along your arms and torso.

[COMPLETE STRETCH]

As the gust subsides, gently un-stretch and release your tension.

[PAUSE]

You end your stretch and a wave crashes against the shore, releasing its energy into the sand.

[PAUSE]

The sun overhead bathes you in an ocean of peaceful clear light.

[PAUSE]

The wind begins to grow more gentle.

[PAUSE]

Even more easily than before, slowly reach up and stretch. Stretch all the way, barely moving a leaf.

[PAUSE]

Gently return to your upright posi-tion, as a wave quietly releases it ten-sion against the shore. At the end of the stretch, let yourself settle into stillness in the warm sun.

[COMPLETE STRETCH. REPEAT FOR NECK, FACE, AND LEGS.]

Let yourself enjoy this relaxation. You have the capacity within for cre-ating peace and calm. Let your mind attend to the good sensations you have created.

[PAUSE]

The waves have settled into quiet ripples lapping against the shore.
[PAUSE]

As you let yourself sink deeper into a pleasant state of inner calm, very slowly and easily rock back and forth to the easy rhythm of the waves.
[PAUSE 10 SECONDS.]

Let your movements be so gentle that they barely stir the air.
[PAUSE 10 SECONDS.]

You have few cares or concerns as you attend only to this rocking motion.
[PAUSE]

Quietly overhead, the sun continues to touch all with its delicate and gentle rays.
[PAUSE]

The wind becomes completely quiet, and the ocean is still.
[PAUSE]

Let your body become completely motionless as you settle into a deeper calm.
[PAUSE]

It is good to let your mind center on the warm sun against your skin. It reminds you that you can trust your innermost thoughts and feelings.
[PAUSE]

Whenever your mind wanders, that's OK.
[PAUSE]

Gently return to the sun as it bathes you in peaceful life-giving light.
[PAUSE]

This is your meditation focus for the next five minutes.
[PAUSE 5 MINUTES.]

Gently let go of what you are attending to. Attend to the sounds around you.

What do you hear?

[PAUSE]

Slowly open your eyes, letting light in bit by bit.

[PAUSE]

What do you see?

And take a deep breath and stretch.

This completes our relaxation exercise.

A Movement Exercise

Goal: Preparing for an assertive encounter

Unifying idea: Flowing with the present.

Attend to the muscles in your right hand and fingers.

Make a tight fist now.

Attend to the feelings of tightness.

By holding and keeping your thoughts and feelings to yourself, you create needless tension.

And let go.

Feel the flow of energy as you release the resistance you have created.

There is nothing for you to do but attend to the good feelings of relaxation.

Notice the difference between tension and relaxation.

And now, slowly, smoothly, and gently open the fingers of your right hand.

Let them stretch more and more completely. Imagine energy flowing down your hands, into your fingers, and out of your fingertips.

As your fingers open, you open to the world. As energy is released, slowly, smoothly, and gently release your stretch.

Very gently return your fingers to their original resting position.

Take your time, let yourself flow easily and gracefully.

[REPEAT PMR AND STRETCHING CYCLES FOR ARMS, BACK, NECK, SHOULDERS, AND FACE.]

Good. Continue attending to your right hand. While remaining still, let warm and tingling sensations spread from your hands to your fingers.

Let these feelings slowly dissolve feelings of tension and carry it through your fingertips.

Notice the good feelings you can create by not blocking the flow of the moment.

It's okay to be open to your feelings. They are good and can be trusted. You do not have to hold them to yourself.

For the next three minutes quietly attend to the warmth and tingling in your hands and fingers.

A Children's Relaxation

Goal: To relax in the middle of the day
Unifying idea: "The Little Train That Could" (let go)

Imagine you are an old steam engine taking a long trip into the countryside. All the passengers have been seated. You're about ready to leave the station. Friendly crowds wave to you and you smile and wave back. The moment is alive with energy and excitement.

As steam begins to build in your giant engine, take in a deep breath and tighten up your shoulders. Let the tension build. Hold the tension. And relax and exhale. As you release a puff of steam, imagine giving all your cars a gentle tug. The train begins to move and coast along the tracks. You can begin to relax and let your muscles become more and more limp. There is nothing you have to do but coast along the tracks.

Now it is time to move a little bit faster. Take in a breath and tighten up your shoulders. Let the tension build. And let go, tugging your cars again. The train coasts along and you relax. Notice the good feelings as you become more calm.

[PMR EXERCISES ARE RE-PEATED FOR THE BACK, NECK, FACE, ARMS, AND LEGS.]

You are now rolling through the countryside. You can relax even more because the train is moving on its own. The engine chugs smoothly and evenly, and little clouds of steam float into the sky.

Let your breathing become smooth and easy.

Quietly open your lips, and slowly exhale. See if you can make the flow of steam so smooth that it barely stirs the air. With every outgoing breath, let yourself relax. As you move along the track, you move further from the worries of the day, deeper into the peaceful countryside. There is nothing you have to do but breathe slowly and evenly.

You have traveled deep into the country. All the things that cause trouble for you are far in the distance. The track has become smoother and you can barely hear or feel the chugging of the engine. Your breathing is very calm and even. Restful hills roll past, covered with soft green grass, trees, and an occasional pond. Contented sheep graze lazily. You can feel the warm, friendly sun against your skin. It feels good and comfortable. Look at the world silently flowing past. Notice all the wonderful relaxing things you can see and hear. [CONTINUE WITH IMAGERY FOR 3 MINUTES.]

The sun is beginning to set. As evening comes, the colors outside become gray. A soft blanket of silence covers everything. All you feel is the peaceful rocking of the train and your breath slowly flowing in and out. Let yourself easily rock, like a train rocking on the tracks. Let each rocking motion be so quiet that it can barely be noticed. For the next few remaining minutes, quietly attend to your rocking motion, slowly back and forth. Whenever your mind wanders, that's okay. Gently rock back and forth. That is all you need to attend to. It can be good to take a rest from the problems of the day. A rest can give you more power to do the things you want to do. Let yourself relax and rock for the next few minutes.

A Creativity Exercise

Goal: Facilitate idea generation
Unifying idea: The black stone
Take in a full, deep breath and quietly exhale.

It is time to put aside effort and deliberate thought.

You are about to embark on a journey into your mind.

Once again, take in a compete breath, and exhale, this time a bit more gently.
[PAUSE 10 SECONDS.]

You will have an opportunity to ask a question important to you and silently let answers come from an inner source of creativity.
[PAUSE]

Continue to breathe fully and easily. Let each breath become increasingly calm.
[PAUSE 10 SECONDS.]

Take your time. There is no need to hurry. Let yourself become centered for your inner journey.
[PAUSE 1 MINUTE.]

Imagine you are at the edge of a forest. The air is calm with anticipation and the sun waits silently overhead. Occasionally, the song of a bird echoes into silence.
[PAUSE 10 SECONDS.]

In front of you is the opening of a cave. You slowly approach and gaze inside. A long flight of granite stairs descends into darkness.

[PAUSE]

Here is where your journey begins. Even though the cave is dark, you feel reassured. Calmly and confidently, you begin your descent. One step at a time.

[PAUSE]

A quiet voice starts counting down, from five to one. With each number, you gently breathe in and out and descend a step. With each number, you let yourself become more centered, more open to the possibilities ahead.

[PAUSE]

Five . . .

You breathe, and take one step.

[PAUSE]

Four . . .

[PAUSE]

It is safe to let yourself be completely free from the constraints of the outside world.

[PAUSE]

Three . . .

[PAUSE]

Your mind becomes increasingly clear.

[PAUSE]

Two . . .

[PAUSE]

The cares of the outside world seem so distant.

[PAUSE]

One . . .

[PAUSE]

At the end of the stairs you encounter a mysterious dark shining stone, as clear as a mirror, reaching from floor to roof.

[PAUSE]

Let your attention become centered on the darkness ahead. It almost seems as though you were looking into the infinite expanse of space. The stone seems deep with mystery. It seems alive.
[PAUSE]

Quietly attend to the stone and gently ask your question. And simply wait.
[PAUSE]

Say nothing. Do nothing. Expect nothing.
[PAUSE]

A creative source deep within holds the potential for answering your questions.
[PAUSE]

Attend to what the stone has to reveal to you, in whatever way or form it desires.
[PAUSE 10 SECONDS.]

And whenever the stone responds, you acknowledge by nodding silently.
[PAUSE]

Continue attending, without thinking or analyzing any response.
[PAUSE 10 SECONDS.]

Whenever your mind wanders, that's OK. Gently return.
[PAUSE]

This is your focus for the next ten minutes.
[PAUSE 10 MINUTES.]

Gently let go of what you are attending to.
[PAUSE]

Slowly acknowledge the stone and turn away.
[PAUSE]

You slowly begin climbing the stairs, step by step.

One . . .

You climb closer to the surface.

Two . . .

You can hear the noises of the world outside.

Three . . .

Feeling quiet and peaceful, you approach the opening.

Four . . .

All around you is bright with sunlight.

Five . . .

Gently open your eyes.

Take a deep breath.

This completes our relaxation sequence.

TABLE 4.1   Relaxation Scripting Worksheet

1. What is your client's relaxation goal?

2. What is your client's unifying idea?

3. What specific relaxation exercises does your client want to include?

PMR	AT	Breathing
❑ Hand	❑ Heavy	❑ Body arch breathing
❑ Hand and arm	❑ Warm	❑ Bowing and breathing
❑ Arm and side	❑ Heart	❑ Bowing, stretching
❑ Back	❑ Breathing	❑ Stomach squeeze
❑ Shoulders	❑ Solar plexus	❑ Stomach touch
❑ Back of neck	❑ Forehead	❑ Book breathing
❑ Face		❑ Inhaling—nose
❑ Front of neck		❑ Exhaling—lips
❑ Stomach and chest		❑ Deep breaths
❑ Legs/thighs		❑ Focused breathing
❑ Feet		

Stretching	Insight imagery	Meditation
❑ Hand	❑ _____	❑ Body sense
❑ Hand and arm		❑ Rocking
❑ Arm and side		❑ Breathing
❑ Back		❑ Mantra
❑ Shoulders		❑ Visual image
❑ Back of neck		❑ External image
❑ Face		❑ Sound
❑ Front of neck		❑ Mindfulness
❑ Stomach and chest		
❑ Legs/thighs		
❑ Feet		

TABLE 4.1 *(continued)*

4. On a word processor, write down the explicit (word-by-word) instructions for each exercise in the order your client prefers. Each phrase gets a separate line. For example, here is the right way of typing a yoga arm stretch:

Slowly let your right arm begin to rise.

Let it rise higher and higher in the air.

Let it rise like the wing of a bird

Or the hand of the clock.

Let it stretch all the way to the sky.

Stretch more and more.

Hold the stretch.

Feel the good sensations of stretching.

Notice how each idea is on a separate line. This simplifies the job of adding ideas and phrases—simply insert them between lines. Here is the wrong way of typing the same stretch:

Slowly let your right arm begin to rise. Let it rise higher and higher in the air. Let it rise like the wing of a bird or the hand of the clock.
Let it stretch all the way to the sky. Stretch more and more.
Hold the stretch. Feel the good sensations of stretching.

If you do not have a word processor, write each phrase on a 3-by-5-inch card. Put additional phases on separate cards, again one phrase per card. Insert these revisions and elaborations into your stack of instructions.

5. Now add phrases that suggest your client's unifying idea. Add one suggestion no more than once every four lines.
6. Add imagery and meditation elaborations.
7. Insert words and phrases to deepen relaxation.
8. Revise instructions to enhance coherence.
9. Add anticipations of setback.
10. Add reinforcing phrases.
11. Add anticipations of setback, reinforcements, pauses and silences, and termination segment.

TABLE 4.5   Extended Relaxation Word List

_____ 1. ABSORBED	_____ 31. FUN	_____ 61. REFRESHED
_____ 2. ACCEPTED	_____ 32. GLORIOUS	_____ 62. RESTED
_____ 3. ACCEPTING	_____ 33. GLOWING	_____ 63. RESTORED
_____ 4. ASLEEP	_____ 34. HAPPY	_____ 64. REVERENT
_____ 5. ASSURED	_____ 35. HARMONIOUS	_____ 65. SELFLESS
_____ 6. AT EASE	_____ 36. HEALING	_____ 66. SENSUOUS
_____ 7. AWAKE	_____ 37. HEAVY	_____ 67. SILENT
_____ 8. AWARE	_____ 38. HOPEFUL	_____ 68. SIMPLE
_____ 9. BEAUTIFUL	_____ 39. INDIFFERENT	_____ 69. SINKING
_____ 10. BLESSED	_____ 40. INFINITE	_____ 70. SOOTHED
_____ 11. CALM	_____ 41. INSPIRED	_____ 71. SPEECHLESS
_____ 12. CAREFREE	_____ 42. JOYFUL	_____ 72. SPIRITUAL
_____ 13. CHILDLIKE	_____ 43. KNOWING	_____ 73. SPONTANEOUS
_____ 14. CLEAR	_____ 44. LAID BACK	_____ 74. STRENGTHENED
_____ 15. COMPLETE	_____ 45. LIGHT	_____ 75. THANKFUL
_____ 16. CONFIDENT	_____ 46. LIMP	_____ 76. TIMELESS
_____ 17. CONTENTED	_____ 47. LIQUID	_____ 77. TINGLING
_____ 18. CREATIVE	_____ 48. LOOSE	_____ 78. TRUSTING
_____ 19. DELIGHTED	_____ 49. LOVED	_____ 79. UNAFRAID
_____ 20. DETACHED	_____ 50. LOVING	_____ 80. UNTROUBLED
_____ 21. DISSOLVING	_____ 51. MYSTERIOUS	_____ 81. WARM
_____ 22. DISTANT	_____ 52. MYSTICAL	_____ 82. WHOLE
_____ 23. DROWSY	_____ 53. OPTIMISTIC	_____ 83. WONDERFUL
_____ 24. ENERGIZED	_____ 54. PASSIVE	
_____ 25. FASCINATED	_____ 55. PATIENT	NEW WORDS:
_____ 26. FAR AWAY	_____ 56. PEACEFUL	
_____ 27. FLOATING	_____ 57. PLAYFUL	
_____ 28. FOCUSED	_____ 58. PLEASED	
_____ 29. FORGETTING	_____ 59. PRAYERFUL	
_____ 30. FREE	_____ 60. QUIET	

5

Brief Relaxation Training

Brief Relaxation Training (BRT) is an accelerated version of ABC Relaxation Training. It is perhaps the most useful approach to relaxation presented in this book, one that is a true test of a relaxation trainer's proficiency. Considerable practice is required before trainers can present BRT fluently. (To facilitate mastery, the BRT protocol is parallel to the Grand Tour protocol). But the rewards can be great. BRT enables the trainer to develop and present an individualized relaxation program in less than an hour (and in some cases, a few minutes). In this brief period of time, the trainer assesses client relaxation needs, demonstrates key exercises, and presents an improvised script. A trainer who masters BRT has at his or her disposal a tool of considerable versatility.

THE BRT PROCEDURE

Brief relaxation training involves three general steps.

Step 1. You demonstrate and your client tries sample exercises from the following:

Progressive Muscle Relaxation
Autogenic Training
Yogaform Stretching
Breathing
Imagery
Meditation

The number of exercises sampled depends on how much time is available. If a full hour is available, present the entire script described here.

If a half-hour is available, demonstrate only the first 2 or 3 exercises from each.

When presenting sample exercises, continuously assess client reactions and preferences. I suggest using a head shake signal system in which you (1) demonstrate an exercise while the client practices; (2) ask the client to shake their head "yes," "no," or simply shrug their shoulders to indicate if they preferred, did not prefer, or are uncertain about the exercise just sampled; and (3) record the client's response in the appropriate table. For PMR, yogaform stretching, and meditation, whenever a client shakes their head "no" for three exercises, abandon the approach and proceed to the next approach. A highly skilled trainer can dispense with this signal system and rely of client nonverbal body cues to determine which exercises to pursue, elaborate upon, or abandon.

Step 2. Once exercises have been sampled, present the client with a list of preferred exercises. You and your client select which exercises to include in the final sequence. Present a list of R-State words and R-Belief affirmations and ask the client to select which they would like included.

Step 3. Present the entire final relaxation sequence to the client, or make a tape, integrating exercises, R-State words and R-Belief affirmations.

Here is the Brief Relaxation Training script:

THE BRT SCRIPT

Rationale

Today we are going to have fun exploring a variety of relaxation exercises. What we will be doing is not hypnosis. You will be in charge. All you have to do is enjoy each exercise as I present the instructions.

First, what is your reason for wanting to learn relaxation? What is your relaxation goal? [RECORD ON TABLE 5.1 AT END OF CHAPTER]

About how many minutes in length do you want your exercise to be? [RECORD]

Here is the procedure we will use. As I give instructions for exercises, from time to time I may ask if you like the approach I am giving. If you do, simply nod your head "yes," like this [DEMONSTRATE]. If not, nod "no" [DEMONSTRATE]. If you are not sure, slightly shrug your shoulders [DEMONSTRATE]. When we are through I will direct you in an exercise sequence that combines the exercises you liked best.

One of our concluding exercises involves quietly attending to a candle flame, which I will light now. [LIGHT CANDLE]

At this time sit upright in a comfortable position. Rest your feet comfortably on the floor. We are now ready to begin.

Demonstrations

Our tour of exercises comes in two parts. First we will let go of our tensions and take a vacation from the cares and concerns of the world. We will let ourselves sink deep into a pleasant and safe relaxation place, a comfortable place where we need to do nothing and can forget the world.

Progressive Muscle Relaxation

[DEMONSTRATE THE FOLLOWING PMR EXERCISES. NOTE WHICH WERE LIKED AND NOT LIKED WHEN YOU ASK CLIENT TO NOD HEAD. CHECK EXERCISES IN TABLE 5.2. WHEN THREE EXERCISES ARE NOT ACCEPTED, PROCEED TO THE AUTOGENIC EXERCISES

1. SHOULDER SQUEEZE
2. ARM SQUEEZE [RIGHT]
3. BACK OF NECK SQUEEZE
4. FACE SQUEEZE
5. FRONT OF NECK SQUEEZE
6. LEG [RIGHT] SQUEEZE
7. IF THE CLIENT REALLY LIKES THESE, YOU MAY ADD TWO OR THREE MORE.]

Specific PMR Instructions for Beginning Instructors

Shoulders
We begin by focusing on the shoulder muscles.
Squeeze your shoulders, now.
Create a nice good shrug.
Let the feelings of tightness grow.
And let go.

Let the tension flow out.
Let your tension begin to unwind.
Let the muscles begin to smooth out.
Let the muscles become more deeply relaxed.
Did you like this exercise? Yes or no? [RECORD]

Shoulder [Repeat]
Again, squeeze the shoulder muscles, now.
Let the muscles get nice and hard.
Let the feelings of tightness grow.
And let go.
Let the muscles go limp.
There is nothing you have to do.
Let feelings of tension dissolve.
Did you like this exercise? Yes or no? [RECORD]

Right Arm
This time focus on your right arm.
Squeeze your lower and upper arm together, now.
Press tighter and tighter.
Notice the feelings of tension.
And let go.
Let the tension go.
Let the rest of your body remain relaxed.
The tension melts away.
Let the muscles become more deeply relaxed.

Right Arm [Repeat]
Again, squeeze your lower and upper arm together, now.
Don't tense up so it hurts.
Tense up only the muscles of the arm.
And let go.
Let your muscles go limp.
As you relax, your muscles become more loose.
You sink deeper into relaxation.
Far away from the cares of the world.
Did you like this exercise? [RECORD]

Back of Neck
Focus on the muscles in the back of the neck.
Gently tilt your head back and gently press the back
   of Your head against your neck, now.
Tighten up the muscles.
Squeeze the muscles more and more.
And let go.

Let the muscles become more deeply relaxed.
Let your entire body become loose and limp.
Let yourself sink deeper and deeper into relaxation.
Let yourself forget the tensions and cares of the world.

Back of Neck [Repeat]
Once again, tighten up the back of the neck, now.
Tighter and tighter.
Tense up only the muscles of back of the neck.
And let go.
Let the tension flow away.
Your muscles feel relaxed and soothed.
As you sink far away from the cares of the world.
Did you like this exercise? [RECORD]

Face
This time focus on the muscles of your face.
Squeeze them altogether, now.
Squeeze your jaws, tongue, lip, nose, eyes, eyebrows, and forehead . . . all together. Squeeze your entire face together.
Let the feelings of tightness grow.
And let go.
Feel calm and relaxed.
Let the tension smooth out.
You begin to feel more and more calm.
As you relax, you feel more at ease.

Face [Repeat]
Once again, tighten up the muscles of the face, now.
Take care not to tense up too much.
Tense up only the muscles of the face.
And let go.
Let the tension go.
Let the tension flow out.
Let tension smooth out.
Let yourself forget the tensions and cares of the world.
Did you like this exercise? [RECORD]

Front of Neck
Focus on the muscles of the neck.
Bow your head and gently press your chin down to your chest, now.
Tighten up the muscles.

Let the tension grow.
And let go.
Let tension begin to melt into liquid.
Let the rest of your body remain relaxed.
Let yourself sink deeper and deeper into relaxation.
Like a tight wad of paper, slowly opening up.

Front of Neck [Repeat]
Again, tighten up the front of the neck, now.
Hold the tension as if you were wringing it out.
Create a good feeling of tension.
And let go.
Let the muscles become more deeply relaxed.
Let your muscles go limp.
Let the muscles begin to smooth out.
There is nothing you have to do.
Did you like this exercise? [RECORD]

Right Leg
Focus on the muscles in your right leg.
Tense the muscles in the leg, now [push your leg against
    the leg or back of your chair . . . or press your leg
    tightly against the other leg].
Tighten up the muscles.
Let the tension grow.
And let go.
Relax.
Let yourself feel more at ease.
Your muscles become more and more heavy, as you sink
    deep into relaxation.

Right Leg [Repeat]
Again, tighten up the right leg, now.
Let the feelings of tightness grow.
Let the tension feel satisfying and complete.
And let go.
Let your entire body go completely limp.
Let your whole body relax.
As you forget the cares of the world.
Did you like this exercise? Yes or no? [RECORD]
Please let go of what you are attending to. We are ready
    to move on.

Autogenic Training

[GIVE AUTOGENIC WARMTH/HEAVINESS EXERCISE.]

Specific Instructions for Autogenic Training

Let yourself sink into a comfortable state of relax-
   ation, far away from the cares of the world. This time
   is just for you, you can forget the problems of the
   day.
Simply think the words, "hands and arms, very heavy."
There is no need for you to achieve any effect.
[PAUSE 5 SECONDS]
Hands and arms are very heavy, like gravity is pulling
   them towards the earth.
[PAUSE 5 SECONDS]
Like a magnet is pulling tension away.
[PAUSE 5 SECONDS]
Arms and legs getting heavy.
[PAUSE 5 SECONDS]
Gravity pulling them down.
[PAUSE 5 SECONDS]
Feel the heavy weight as your arms and legs sink.
[PAUSE 5 SECONDS]
Heavier and heavier.
[PAUSE 5 SECONDS]
Entire body, more and more heavy.
[PAUSE]
Let yourself sink into a distant state of pleasant
   relaxation.
[PAUSE]
There is nothing you have to do.
[PAUSE 5 SECONDS]
Let the words, go over and over like an echo.
[PAUSE]
Arms and legs very heavy. Very heavy. Very heavy.
[PAUSE]
There is nothing you have to do.
[PAUSE]
Let tension sink away.

[PAUSE]
Let gravity pull tension away.
[PAUSE]
As you forget your cares and concerns
[PAUSE]
You become more calm and relaxed.
[PAUSE]
More quiet.
[PAUSE]
Entire body, very heavy. Very heavy. Very heavy.
[PAUSE 5 SECONDS]
Your arms become more and more loose and limp.
[PAUSE]
As tension sinks away.
[PAUSE]
Like a magnet pulling tension away.
[PAUSE]
Arms and legs are very heavy.
[PAUSE]
Entire body very heavy.
[PAUSE]
Arms and legs are very heavy.
Let yourself sink into a pleasant state of relaxation.
Far, far away from the cares of the world.
Very distant and detached, as if nothing seems to
   matter.
Very good. Let me know if you liked this exercise. Yes
   or no. [RECORD]
Please let go of what you are attending to. We are ready
   to move on.

We have just completed our first set of exercises. How do you feel?
We will now continue our tour of relaxation by trying a different set
of exercises. These will help you feel relaxed and refreshed. With
a clear and peaceful mind, we will let ourselves become open to
and enjoy interesting new worlds of relaxation.

Yogaform Stretching

[CONTINUE WITH THE FOLLOWING YOGAFORM STRETCHES.
WHEN THREE EXERCISES ARE NOT ACCEPTED, PROCEED
TO THE BREATHING EXERCISES

1. ARM EXTEND AND STRETCH
1. ARM TO SIDE AND CIRCLE UP STRETCH
2. BACK STRETCH
3. BACK OF NECK STRETCH
4. FACE STRETCH
5. FRONT OF NECK STRETCH
6. IF THE CLIENT REALLY LIKES THESE, YOU MAY ADD TWO
   OR THREE MORE.]

Specific Instructions for Yogaform Stretching

Arm Extend and Stretch
Now move to your right arm.
Slowly, smoothly, and gently slide you hand down
   your leg.
Extend your arm farther and farther.
Reach out and extend your arm in front of you.
Very gracefully, like you are balancing a feather on
   each Hand.
And hold the stretch and become aware of the
   sensations.
Then slowly, smoothly, and gently release the stretch.
Gently rest your hand on your leg and slide your arm
   back to its resting position.
Take your time.
Slowly and gently unstretch your arm.
Do you want to include this exercise? [RECORD]
Arm to Side Circle up and Stretch
Now let both your arms fall limply to your sides.
Slowly, smoothly, and gently circle your right arm and
   hand up and away from your body like the hand of a
   clock or the wing of a bird.
Let your arm extend straight, and circle higher and
   higher.
Let it circle to the sky.
And they circle your arm over your head so your hand
   points to the other side . . . And arch your body as
   you reach and point farther and farther, like a tree
   arching in the wind.
Become aware of the invigorating feelings of
   stretching.

Now gently and easily,
Like the hand of a clock or the wing of a bird circle
   your arm back over your head . . . to your side
Finally to the resting position.
And let your arm hang.
Do you want to include this exercise? [RECORD]

Back Stretch

Now focus your attention on your back, below your
   shoulders.
Slowly, smoothly, and gently relax and bow over.
Let your arms hang limply.
Let your head fall forward, as you bow forward farther
   and farther in your chair.
Do not force yourself to bow over . . . let gravity
   pull your body toward your knees . . . farther and
   farther.
It's ok to take a short breath if you need to.
Feel the stretch along the back.
Let gravity pull your body forward, as far as it will go.
Then gently and easily sit up.
Take your time.
Inch by inch, straighten up your body.
Until you are seated comfortably in an upright
   position.
Do you want to include this exercise? [RECORD]

Back of Neck Stretch

Now, while sitting erect, let your head tilt easily
   toward your chest.
Try not to force it down.
Simply let gravity pull your head down.
Farther and farther.
Focus on the stretch in the back of your neck.
The refreshing and renewing energy it releases.
As the force of gravity easily and slowly pulls your
   head down.
When you are ready, gently and easily lift your head.
Lift it until it is again comfortably upright.
Should we include this exercise? [RECORD]

Face Stretch

Now attend to the muscles of your face.

Slowly, smoothly, and gently open your jaws, mouth, and eyes while lifting your eyebrows.

Open wide.

Feel every muscle of your face stretch more and more.

Hold the stretch.

Then gently and easily release the stretch.

Let the muscles smooth out as they relax.

Let your face settle into a comfortable position.

Do you want to include this exercise? [RECORD]

Front of Neck Stretch

Now, like before, let your head tilt, this time backward.

Let gravity pull your head back, but not too far, just enough to feel the stretch.

Do not force it back.

Let gravity do the work for you as it pulls the heavy weight of your head back farther and farther.

Gently and slightly open your mouth, and let your head relax and fall back.

Focus your mind on the front of the neck stretch as it stretches.

Gently hold the stretch.

Then gently and easily lift your head.

Gradually return it to its upright position

take your time. There is no need to hurry.

Shall we include this exercise? [RECORD]

Please let go of what you are attending to. We are ready to move on.

Breathing

[CONTINUE WITH THE FOLLOWING BREATHING EXERCISES. RECORD PREFERENCES.

1. BREATHING IN WITH SNIFFS
2. BREATHING OUT THROUGH LIPS
3. DEEP BREATHING]

Specific Breathing Exercise Instructions

Breathing in with Sniffs

As you breathe in, imagine you are sniffing a very delicate flower.

Let the flow of breath into your nose be as smooth and
gentle as possible, so you barely rustle a petal.

Take a full breath.

And relax, letting yourself breathe out slowly and
naturally, without effort.

Continue breathing this way, breathing in and out,
quietly and evenly at your own pace.

Calmly focus on the clear inner calm that comes when
you breathe in a way that is slow, full, and even.

Notice the refreshing and energizing rush of air as it
quietly moves in and out of your lungs.

See how far you can follow the inward flow of air.

Can you feel it move past your nostrils?

Can you feel the air in the passages of your nose?

Can you feel the renewing and refreshing air flow into
your body?

Take your time.

Breathe easily and fully.

Let yourself be fully aware of your breathing.

[PAUSE]

Do you want to include this exercise? [RECORD]

Breathing out Through Lips

Take a slow deep breath and pause.

And breathe out slowly though your lips, as if you were
blowing at a candle flame just enough to make it
flicker, but not go out. Continue breathing out, emptying all the air from your stomach and chest.

Then breathe in through your nose.

Continue breathing this way making the stream of air
that passes through your lips as you exhale as
smoothly and gently as possible.

Let tension flow out with every breath.

Let the gentle movement of air dissolve any feelings
of tension you might have.

Focus on the easy flow of air in as it refreshes and
renews.

Let each breath fill you with peace and calm energy.

Let yourself breathe fully and evenly.

Should we include this exercise? [RECORD]

Deep Breathing

Let yourself breathe easily and naturally.

When you are ready, take in a full deep breath, filling your lungs and abdomen with good, refreshing air.

And when you are ready, relax.

And slowly let the air flow out, very smoothly and gently.

And now, just continue breathing normally for a while.

Do not attempt to force yourself to breathe in any particular way.

Just let the air come in and out on its own.

[PAUSE 10 SECONDS]

And, again, when you are ready, take in a full deep breath.

Filling your lungs, with good, energizing air. Feel the calm and strength it brings.

And, when ready, gently and smoothly exhale.

Then resume breathing in a normal way, easily in and out.

[PAUSE 10 SECONDS]

How was that? [RECORD] Please let go of what you are attending to. We are ready to move on.

Imagery

Specific Imagery Script

We are going to relax with a peaceful fantasy. Imagine you are in a very relaxing place. Perhaps you are by a lake or ocean, or in a forest or garden, or even a quiet cabin. It doesn't matter where you are. Imagine all of the details. Perhaps you can see the peaceful sky and clouds. Maybe there are clouds. Or rushing water. Can you feel the cool refreshing air, or the warm sun on your skin? Perhaps you can hear the rustle of leaves or grass, or maybe the flow of water, or the quiet songs of birds. Can you smell the relaxing fragrances around you? Imagine this place with all your senses.

[PAUSE 60 SECONDS]

Indicate if you would like some imagery in your exercise. [RECORD]

**[THE FOLLOWING ADVANCED IMAGERY EXERCISE MAY BE
ADDED BY EXPERIENCED INSTRUCTORS, IF THE CLIENT EN-
JOYED THE PREVIOUS SENSE IMAGERY]**

Optional Additional Imagery Script

Let us continue with our fantasy.
This image is actually a story of a journey. In it you
   go to a special place, one that has a message of calm
   and peace for you. There is nothing for you to do or
   think about. Simply relax, and enjoy the journey.
Imagine you are traveling a long distance. Perhaps you
   are in a boat, train, even balloon, it doesn't matter.
You see many wonderful things coming and going. The
   sky. The scenery outside. You can feel the sun and
   fresh air. You can hear the wind, and smell the fresh
   fragrance of trees.
[PAUSE]
You come to the end of your journey. It is an outdoor
   nature setting.
[PAUSE]
It is a wonderful and beautiful place, filled with mys-
   tery and wonder.
You can see green all around—trees, grass, flowers.
   The sky above is a clear blue.
You can feel a gentle breeze against your skin.
And the warm sun.
You hear the wind blowing through the trees or grass.
Perhaps you hear the song of a distant bird.
It is a wonderful and relaxing place.
And in this place you discover a clear pond.
Its surface is very still, like a perfect mirror re-
   flect the blue sky and clouds above. In the distance
   you notice a person walking, someone who is very wise.
   This can be a religious leader, a philosopher,
   teacher, or someone in your life.
This setting has a special message for you. It is a
   special message of calm and peace. This message can

come to you in many ways. Perhaps the message will
appear reflected in the surface of the pond. Perhaps
the person in the distance has a message to say to
you. The message can be anything. It can even be something as simple as your beautiful surroundings, that
create feelings of calm and peace.
And there is absolutely nothing you have to do.
Simply and calmly attend without trying to figure any-
thing out.
If thoughts come to mind, that's fine. Simply and gen-
tly put them aside, and continue attending.
If you find yourself starting to figure things out,
that's fine.
Simply put your thoughts aside, and calmly attend to
the setting. That is all you need to do.
[PAUSE]
There is nothing to figure out.
This is a place of calm and peace.
[WAIT 1 MINUTE]
Gently let go of what you are thinking of.
Do you think you would like to relax with an imagery
story?
[RECORD] Please let go of what you are attending to. We
are now ready to move on to our final set of exercises.

Meditation

[1. ROCKING MEDITATION
2. BREATHING MEDITATION
3. MANTRA MEDITATION
4. MEDITATION ON A VISUAL IMAGE
5. MEDITATION ON AN EXTERNAL IMAGE.
RECORD PREFERENCES. WHEN THREE MEDITATIONS ARE
NOT ACCEPTED, CONTINUE TO THE NEXT SECTION.]

Specific Meditation Instructions

Meditation is a very simple exercise. In fact, the instructions can be said in two sentences: calmly attend to a simple stimulus. Calmly return your
attention after every distraction . . . again and

again and again. In this exercise we will be exploring several meditations. You will have a chance to select which work best for you.

Rocking Meditation.

Think of all the times in life you have found the gentle movement of *rocking* very calm and soothing. You might be on a rowboat in a lake, gently bobbing back and forth as waves gently lap against you. Perhaps you are in a rocking chair on a porch. You are at peace. Nothing is on your mind. You gently rock back and forth, again and again. Perhaps you are resting on a hammock, swinging very gently. You might even be rocking a small child in your arms. There is indeed something very soothing and meditative, about simple rocking.

At this time let yourself begin to rock back and forth in your chair.

[PAUSE]

Let each movement become more and more gentle and easy. Let yourself rock effortlessly. Let your body move on its own, in its own way, at its own speed. All you have to do is simply attend.

[PAUSE]

Let each movement become more and more subtle so that someone watching would barely notice you are rocking. All you have to do is quietly attend to the repetitive back and forth movement, like rocking on a boat or a rocking chair. Every time your mind wanders, that's okay; gently return to your rocking motion.

For the next minute or so, let your rocking become barely noticeable. And quietly attend.

[PAUSE 90 SECONDS]

Gently let go of what you are attending to. Meditation is very simple. If your mind wandered, that's ok. If you are distracted, that's ok.

And now let me know if you liked rocking meditation?

[RECORD]

Breathing Meditation.

We move on. Take in a full breath, and relax. Let your breathing continue on its own in a way that is free and easy. There is nothing you have to do. Simply attend to flow of breath, in and out. And return your attention whenever your mind wanders or is distracted.

[PAUSE 90 SECONDS]

Gently let go of what you are attending to. Did you like breathing meditation?

[RECORD]

Mantra Meditation.

We move on. Let the word *peace* come to you like an echo in the distance. Let the word peace repeat over and over and over, at its own pace and volume.

Peace . . . Peace . . . peace.

[PAUSE 90 SECONDS]

Gently let go of what you are attending to.

Did you like this meditation?

[RECORD]

Meditation on a Visual Image.

We are ready to move on again. With your eyes closed, think of the image of a simple spot of light, a candle flame, or a star.

And calmly attend.

And calmly return after every distraction.

[PAUSE 90 SECONDS]

Gently let go of what you are attending to. Did you like this meditation?

[RECORD]

Meditation on an External Image.

This time, slowly open your eyes halfway. Easily gaze on the candle in front of you. Whenever your mind wanders, gently return.

[PAUSE 90 SECONDS]

Gently let go of what your are attending to.

Did you like this meditation?

[RECORD]

RING CHIME OR BELL ONCE. WAIT FOR 1 MINUTE].

We have now finished our tour of relaxation. It is time to select what you want for your relaxation sequence.

Preparation for Dress Rehearsal

Exercise Selection

[GIVE CLIENT THE RELAXATION EXERCISES LIST (TABLE 5.2).
CLIENT THEN DECIDES HOW LONG THE SEQUENCE IS TO BE
(FROM 5 TO 15 MINUTES). EACH EXERCISE SELECTED TAKES
ABOUT ONE MINUTE. CLIENT IS PERMITTED TO SELECT ONLY
THE NUMBER OF EXERCISES APPROPRIATE FOR THE NUM-
BER OF MINUTES SELECTED. NO MORE THAN ONE IMAGERY
AND ONE MEDITATION CAN BE SELECTED (EACH COUNTS
3 MINUTES)].

Optional Imagery Selection

[IF YOUR CLIENT LIKED IMAGERY, GIVE THESE IMAGERY SPE-
CIAL INSTRUCTIONS]:

Sometimes people pick a daydream theme that runs into problems. It might seem fine at first, but has a hidden "booby trap" within.
For example, you might want to think of the lake you visited as a
child, not realizing you nearly drowned in the lake. This painful
thought might arise unexpectedly in your daydream, and spoil your
relaxation. Can you think of any hidden problems in your theme?

[IF PROBLEMS ARE MENTIONED, PICK ANOTHER THEME.]

Now we need to paint the details for your imagery exercise. What
might you see? What might you hear or feel touching your skin?
What might you smell that is relaxing? Let's see if we can think of
some ideas, while I write them down.
[ASK CLIENT FOR AT LEAST 4 OR FIVE SENSE DETAILS FOR
EACH CATEGORY: WHAT IS SEEN, HEARD, FELT, AND
SMELLED. WRITE THEM DOWN ON YOUR RELAXATION EXER-
CISES LIST.]

Relaxation Word and Phrase List

[ONCE CLIENT SELECTS EXERCISES, PRESENT THE RELAX-
ATION WORD AND PHRASE LIST IN TABLES 5.3 AND 5.4 AND
HAVE THEM CHECK OFF WHICH WORDS AND PHRASES THEY
WOULD LIKE YOU TO ADD TO THEIR RELAXATION EXER-
CISES. INTRODUCE WITH THESE INSTRUCTIONS]:

Here is a list of words and phrases people often find relaxing. Please let me know which you find relaxing so I can add them to your final relaxation sequence.

Dress Rehearsal

[ONCE SPECIFIC EXERCISES, RELAXATION WORDS, AND AFFIRMATION PHRASES HAVE BEEN DETERMINED, YOU PROCEED WITH THE DRESS REHEARSAL. THE CLIENT CLOSES HIS OR HER EYES AND PRACTICES AS YOU SPEAK THE INSTRUCTIONS. TO DO THIS YOU MUST HAVE THE RELAXATION EXERCISE LIST AND THE RELAXATION WORD AND PHRASE LISTS IN FRONT OF YOU (TABLES 5.2–5.4). THESE WILL BE YOUR GUIDES. IN SPEAKING THE INSTRUCTIONS, USE THE FOLLOWING GUIDELINES:

• EACH PROGRESSIVE MUSCLE RELAXATION, YOGAFORM STRETCHING EXERCISE, AND BREATHING EXERCISE IS TO BE DONE TWICE.
• PROGRESSIVE MUSCLE RELAXATION AND YOGAFORM STRETCHING EXERCISES DONE ON THE RIGHT SIDE OF THE BODY ARE TO BE ALSO DONE ON THE LEFT SIDE.
• AFTER EVERY TEN RELAXATION PHRASES, INTRODUCE ONE OF THE RELAXATION WORDS THE CLIENT CHECKED FROM THE RELAXATION WORDLIST.
• TWO OR THREE TIMES ADD A FEW WORDS OF REINFORCEMENT, "GOOD, YOU ARE DOING FINE, EXCELLENT."
• TWO OR THREE TIMES ADD A FEW PHRASES OF REASSURANCE, "IF YOUR MIND WANDERS, THAT'S OK, GENTLY RETURN TO THE EXERCISE. . . . IF YOU ARE DISTRACTED, THAT'S FINE, JUST RETURN TO THE EXERCISE."
• AFTER EVERY TWENTY OR SO RELAXATION PHRASES, INTRODUCE A RELAXATION AFFIRMATION PHRASE SUGGESTED BY THE CLIENT. USE YOUR JUDGEMENT. IF THERE IS NO PLACE TO INSERT AN AFFIRMATION PHRASE, INSERT IT AT THE END AS A CLOSING.
• ANY IMAGERY OR MEDITATION SEQUENCE IS TO LAST ONLY 3 MINUTES.

- WHEN YOU GET GOOD AT THIS, TRY TO WEAVE YOUR EXERCISES TOGETHER (INTRODUCING COHERENCE AND INTEGRITY AS SUGGESTED IN TEXT.)
- CLOSE THE EXERCISE WITH "YOU CAN NOW LET GO OF WHAT YOU ARE ATTENDING TO. GENTLY OPEN YOUR EYES BIT BY BIT. TAKE A DEEP BREATH, AND STRETCH. WE HAVE NOW COMPLETED OUR RELAXATION EXERCISE."]

TABLE 5.1   Brief Relaxation Training (BRT) Worksheet

What is your client's relaxation goal?

How long (in minutes) does your client want the relaxation sequence to be?

What specific exercises did your client like? Check these on the Relaxation Exercise List.

TABLE 5.2   Relaxation Exercise List

PMR
_____ Shoulder squeeze
_____ Arm (right) squeeze
_____ Back of neck squeeze
_____ Face squeeze
_____ Front of neck squeeze
_____ Leg (right) squeeze
_____ Others (you may add some if your client really liked these)

AUTOGENIC TRAINING
_____ Hands and arms warm and heavy

FOCUSING AND OPENING UP

YOGAFORM STRETCHING
_____ Arm to front and stretch
_____ Arm to side and circle up stretch
_____ Back stretch
_____ Back of neck stretch
_____ Face stretch
_____ Front of neck stretch
_____ Others

BREATHING
_____ Breathing in with sniffs
_____ Breathing out through lips
_____ Deep breathing

IMAGERY
_____ Imagery topic:
        What is seen:
        What is heard:
        What is touched:
        Fragrances:

MEDITATION:
Preferred meditation:

TABLE 5.3 Relaxation Word List

_____ 1. ABSORBED	_____ 31. FUN	_____ 61. REFRESHED
_____ 2. ACCEPTED	_____ 32. GLORIOUS	_____ 62. RESTED
_____ 3. ACCEPTING	_____ 33. GLOWING	_____ 63. RESTORED
_____ 4. ASLEEP	_____ 34. HAPPY	_____ 64. REVERENT
_____ 5. ASSURED	_____ 35. HARMONIOUS	_____ 65. SELFLESS
_____ 6. AT EASE	_____ 36. HEALING	_____ 66. SENSUOUS
_____ 7. AWAKE	_____ 37. HEAVY	_____ 67. SILENT
_____ 8. AWARE	_____ 38. HOPEFUL	_____ 68. SIMPLE
_____ 9. BEAUTIFUL	_____ 39. INDIFFERENT	_____ 69. SINKING
_____ 10. BLESSED	_____ 40. INFINITE	_____ 70. SOOTHED
_____ 11. CALM	_____ 41. INSPIRED	_____ 71. SPEECHLESS
_____ 12. CAREFREE	_____ 42. JOYFUL	_____ 72. SPIRITUAL
_____ 13. CHILDLIKE	_____ 43. KNOWING	_____ 73. SPONTANEOUS
_____ 14. CLEAR	_____ 44. LAID BACK	_____ 74. STRENGTHENED
_____ 15. COMPLETE	_____ 45. LIGHT	_____ 75. THANKFUL
_____ 16. CONFIDENT	_____ 46. LIMP	_____ 76. TIMELESS
_____ 17. CONTENTED	_____ 47. LIQUID	_____ 77. TINGLING
_____ 18. CREATIVE	_____ 48. LOOSE	_____ 78. TRUSTING
_____ 19. DELIGHTED	_____ 49. LOVED	_____ 79. UNAFRAID
_____ 20. DETACHED	_____ 50. LOVING	_____ 80. UNTROUBLED
_____ 21. DISSOLVING	_____ 51. MYSTERIOUS	_____ 81. WARM
_____ 22. DISTANT	_____ 52. MYSTICAL	_____ 82. WHOLE
_____ 23. DROWSY	_____ 53. OPTIMISTIC	_____ 83. WONDERFUL
_____ 24. ENERGIZED	_____ 54. PASSIVE	
_____ 25. FASCINATED	_____ 55. PATIENT	NEW WORDS:
_____ 26. FAR AWAY	_____ 56. PEACEFUL	
_____ 27. FLOATING	_____ 57. PLAYFUL	
_____ 28. FOCUSED	_____ 58. PLEASED	
_____ 29. FORGETTING	_____ 59. PRAYERFUL	
_____ 30. FREE	_____ 60. QUIET	

TABLE 5.4   Relaxation Phrase List

Belief 1:   View the world with optimism.
            I can be optimistic about my current hassles.
            It is important to be optimistic.
Belief 2:   Accept things the way they are.
            I can accept things as they are.
            There's no need to try to change what can't be changed.
Belief 3:   Be honest with yourself and others.
            I can accept my thoughts and feelings.
            I can be honest and open with my feelings.
Belief 4:   Know when to let go and take it easy.
            Sometimes it is important to simply take it easy.
            It is important to know when to stop trying, let go, and relax.
Belief 5:   Relate to others with love and compassion.
            The love I give and receive is a source of peace and comfort to me.
            It is important to treat people with compassion and understanding.
Belief 6:   Trust the healing wisdom of the body.
            I trust the body's wisdom and healing powers.
            There are sources of strength and healing deep within me.
Belief 7:   Trust God's love and guidance.
            God guides, loves, and comforts me.
            I put myself in God's hands.
Belief 8:   Put your concerns in deeper perspective.
            Life has a purpose greater than my personal wants and desires.
            There's more to life than my personal concerns and worries.

References

Beck, A. T., Ward, C., Mendelson, M., Mock, J., & Erbaugh, J. (1961). An inventory for measuring depression. *Archives of General Psychiatry, 4,* 53–63.

Benson, H. (1975). *The relaxation response.* New York: Morrow.

Bernstein, D. A., & Borkovec, T. D. (1973). *Progressive relaxation training: A manual for the helping professions.* Champaign, IL: Research Press.

Bernstein, D. A., & Carlson, C. R. (1993). Progressive relaxation: Abbreviated methods. In P. M. Lehrer & R. L. Woolfolk (Eds.), *Principles and practice of stress management* (2nd ed., pp. 53–87). New York: Guilford.

Carrington, P. (1978). *Clinical standardized meditation instructor's manual and self-regulating course.* Kendall Park, NJ: Pace Systems.

Davidson, R. J., & Schwartz, G. E. (1976). Psychobiology of relaxation and related states: A multiprocess theory. In D. I. Mostofsky (Ed.), *Behavior control and the modification of physiological activity* (pp. 399–442). Englewood Cliffs, NJ: Prentice Hall.

Derogatis, L. R., & Coons, H. L. (1993). Self-report measures of stress. In L. Goldberger & S. Breznitz (Eds.), *Handbook of stress: Theoretical and clinical aspects* (2nd ed., pp. 200–233). New York: The Free Press.

Fried, R. (1993). The role of respiration in stress and stress control: Toward a theory of stress as a hypoxic phenomenon. In P. M. Lehrer & R. L. Woolfolk (Eds.), *Principles and practice of stress management* (2nd ed., pp. 301–332). New York: Guilford.

Funderburk, J. (1977). *Science studies yoga.* Glenview, IL: Himalayan Institute.

Lazarus, A. A. (1976). *Multimodal behavior therapy.* New York: Springer.

Lazarus, A. A. (1997). *Brief but comprehensive psychotherapy: The multimodal way.* New York: Springer.

Lehrer, P. M., Carr, R., Sargunaraj, D., & Woolfolk, R. L. (1994). Stress management techniques: Are they are equivalent, or do they have specific effects? *Biofeedback and Self-Regulation, 19,* 353–401.

LeShan, L. (1974). *How to meditate.* New York: Bantam.

Ley, R. (1995). Highlights of the 13th International Symposium on Respiratory Psychophysiology Held at the Inaugural Meeting of the International Society for the Advancement of Respiratory Psychophysiology. *Biofeedback and Self-Regulation, 20,* 369–379.

Lichstein, K. (1988). *Clinical relaxation strategies.* New York: Wiley.

Linden, W. (1993). The autogenic training method of J. H. Schultz. In P. M. Lehrer & R. L. Woolfolk (Eds.), *Principles and practice of stress management* (pp. 205–229). New York: Guilford.

McNair, D. M., Lorr, M., & Dropplemann, L. F. (1971). *Profile of Mood States.* San Diego, CA: Educational and Industrial Testing Service.

Patel, C. (1993). Yoga-based therapy. In P. M. Lehrer & R. L. Woolfolk (Eds.), *Principles and practice of stress management* (pp. 89–137). New York: Guilford.

Poppen, R. (1998). *Behavioral relaxation training and assessment* (2nd ed.). New York: Sage.

Radloff, L. S. (1977). The CES-D Scale: A self-report depression scale for research in the general population. *Applied Psychological Measurement, 1,* 385–401.

Smith, J. C. (1989). *Relaxation dynamics: A cognitive-behavioral approach to relaxation.* Champaign, IL: Research Press.

Smith, J. C. (1990). *Cognitive-behavioral relaxation training: A new system of strategies for treatment and assessment.* New York: Springer.

Smith, J. C. (1992). *Spiritual living for a skeptical age.* New York: Insight Press.

Smith, J. C. (1999). *ABC relaxation theory: An attentional behavioral cognitive approach.* New York: Springer.

Smith, J. C., Amutio, A., Anderson, J., & Aria, L. P. (1996). Relaxation: Mapping an uncharted world. *Biofeedback and Self-Regulation, 21,* 63–90.

Smith, J. C. (In press). *ABC Relaxation Research.* New York: Springer.

Spielberger, C. D., Gorsuch, R. C., & Lushene, R. E. (1970). *Manual for the State-Trait Anxiety Inventory.* Palo Alto, CA: Consulting Psychologists Press.

Vahia, N. S., Doongaji, D. R., Jeste, D. V., Ravindranath, S., Kapoor, S. M., & Ardhapurkar, I. (1973). Psychophysiologic therapy based on the concepts of Patanjali. *American Journal of Psychotherapy, 27,* 557–565.

Van Dixhoorn, J. (1994). Significance of breathing awareness and exercise training for recovery after myocardial infarction. In J. G. Carlson, A. R. Seifert, & N. Birbaumer (Eds.), *Clinical applied psychophysiology* (chap. 9). New York: Plenum.

Weinstein, M., & Smith, J. C. (1992). Isometric squeeze relaxation (progressive relaxation) vs. meditation: Absorption and focusing as predictors of state effects. *Perceptual and Motor Skills, 75,* 1263–1271.

Appendix

Smith Relaxation Inventory Series

I am making available five inventories that tap the relaxation variables introduced in this book. The Smith Relaxation States Inventory (SRSI) measures one's immediate level of relaxation and stress. It is appropriate for process studies examining immediate changes during the course of a relaxation activity. The Smith Recalled Relaxation Activity Inventory (SRRAI) asks participants to recall and describe relaxation states associated with a relaxation activity. Much of the research in this book is based on the SRRSI. It is proving to be a highly sensitive measure. The Smith Relaxation Dispositions/Motivations Inventory (SRDMI) measures one's propensity to be relaxed over a two-week period of time (disposition) as well as one's desire to be more relaxed (motivation). Both are appropriate outcome measures for treatment intervention. The Smith Relaxation Beliefs Inventory (SRBI) measures beliefs hypothesized to be conducive to deeper and more generalized relaxation. The Smith Relaxation Concerns Inventory (SRCI) assesses the most frequent goals people have for learning relaxation. The inventories here are tentative versions. For final versions, contact Springer Publishing Company.

INSTRUCTIONS FOR OBTAINING
PERMISSION TO USE

The Smith Relaxation Inventory Series is owned by Springer Publishing Company. It is illegal to use any inventory from this series without prior written permission from the publisher. To acquire permission to copy and use and to receive a scoring key and manual, contact the publisher.

Background Information

Your Gender: ❏ M ❏ F   **Your Age:** _____

Your Annual Income (closest amount):
❏ $10,000 ❏ $20,000 ❏ $30,000 ❏ $40,000 ❏ $50,000 ❏ $60,000 ❏ $70,000
❏ $80,000 ❏ $90,000

Check if you are: ❏ Currently in any type of psychotherapy.

Check if you are taking a prescription psychiatric medication for:
❏ Anxiety ❏ Depression ❏ Other _____

Highest Level of Education:
❏ Some high school ❏ Finished high school ❏ Some college ❏ Finished undergrad
❏ At least some grad school

Are you (optional):
❏ Gay/Lesbian ❏ Bisexual ❏ Heterosexual

Religious Affiliation:
❏ Buddhist ❏ Catholic ❏ Hindu ❏ Jewish ❏ Muslim/Islamic ❏ Protestant
❏ New Age/Yoga/Meditation ❏ None

Family Background:
❏ Upper Class ❏ Middle Class ❏ Blue Collar/Working Class ❏ Poor

Are you:
❏ African American ❏ Hispanic ❏ Caucasian ❏ Native American
❏ Asian/Pacific Islander

How well does the term you chose in the above question describe you?
❏ Not at All ❏ A Little ❏ Moderately ❏ A Lot ❏ Totally

Which best describes your ethnic and cultural heritage?

❏ Africa	❏ South American	❏ Native North American Indian
❏ Chinese	❏ Caribbean Islands	❏ Middle Eastern
❏ Indian/India	❏ Pacific Islands	❏ European
❏ North American	❏ Japanese	❏ Korean ❏ Other Asian

How well does what you chose in the above Question describe you?
❏ Not at All ❏ A Little ❏ Moderately ❏ A Lot ❏ Totally

Were one or both of your parents born in the U.S.?
❏ One ❏ Both ❏ Neither ❏ Don't Know

(continued)

Background Information *(continued)*

Were one or both of your grandparents born in the U.S.?
❑ One ❑ Both ❑ Neither ❑ Don't Know

Many Americans describe themselves as multiethnic, for example, part German, part Italian, and Part Puerto Rican.

Please describe what combinations of ethnic backgrounds are represented in you.

SRRAI

RELAXATION ACTIVITY

PEOPLE DO MANY THINGS FOR *RELAXATION AND RENEWAL*. WE ARE INTER-
ESTED IN WHAT CAN BE DONE *PASSIVELY* IN A RELAXED STANDING,
SEATED, OR RESTING POSITION (*This* **excludes** *hobbies, camping, hiking, taking
trips, dancing, movies, TV, parties, sports, fitness exercises, forms of recreation, sex,
eating, drugs, alcohol, tobacco. We are also excluding activities that involve talking to
or interacting with other people.*) BELOW ARE EXAMPLES OF PASSIVE FORMS
OF RELAXATION AND RENEWAL. PLEASE CHECK HOW MANY **TIMES A
WEEK** you do each activity. Please write your answers in the blanks.

I DO THIS ACTIVITY ___ TIMES A WEEK (FILL IN BLANK BY ITEM)

1. ____	Art / Pictures (Looking at, appreciating)	18. ____	Prayer (alone, not in group)
2. ____	Audio relaxation tapes	19. ____	Prayer (with others, in group)
3. ____	Breathing exercises	20. ____	Progressive muscle relaxation
4. ____	Church/ synagog, temple (attending)	21. ____	Radio, listening to
5. ____	Daydreaming	22. ____	Reading the Bible/ Koran
6. ____	Hatha yoga stretches	23. ____	Reading Fiction
7. ____	Hot tubs / baths	24. ____	Reading (inspirational – not Bible/Koran)
8. ____	Hypnosis (self)	25. ____	Reading Nonfiction
9. ____	Imagery / visualization	26. ____	Reading Poetry
10. ____	Massage	27. ____	Progressive muscle relaxation
11. ____	Meditation, TM	28. ____	Resting in bed
12. ____	Meditation, mantra, not TM	29. ____	Showers, baths
13. ____	Meditation, breathing, Zen, Mindfulness	30. ____	Steam baths
14. ____	Music (Playing for self)	31. ____	Sunbathing
15. ____	Music (Listening to)	32. ____	TV, watching (including video tapes)
16. ____	Nature appreciation	33. ____	Yoga (hatha)
17. ____	Petting pets	34. ____	Walking (leisurely)

(continued)

SRRAI

RELAXATION ACTIVITY
(continued)

Please think about the past two weeks. What was the single MOST REWARDING AND EFFECTIVE passive thing you did for relaxation and renewal? It doesn't have to be any of those listed above. Please describe this in the box below. As much as possible, be specific and detailed:

> MY PASSIVE FORM OF RELAXATION AND RENEWAL
> (DONE IN A RELAXED STANDING, SEATED, OR RESTING POSITION)

How often do you engage in this activity alone, by yourself? How many days out of the week?
❏ Less than 1 day a week ❏ 1 day a week ❏ 2 days ❏ 3 days
❏ 4 days ❏ 5 days ❏ 6 days ❏ 7 days

How often do you engage in this activity in a group, with others?
❏ Less than 1 day a week ❏ 1 day a week ❏ 2 days ❏ 3 days
❏ 4 days ❏ 5 days ❏ 6 days ❏ 7 days

For about how many years and/or months have you engaged in this activity?
_____ Years _____ Months

How skilled are you at this activity? (Skip if not applicable)
❏ 1. Not at all ❏ 2. Slightly ❏ 3. Moderately ❏ 4. Very much

Now, please close your eyes and recall what you've just described in the above box. What was this activity like? What did you experience? On the next page are some phrases that describe experience people often have. Please recall how you felt while engaged in the activity you put in the above box and answer the questions provided.

SRRAI

PLEASE CHECK TO WHAT EXTENT YOU FELT EACH OF THE FOLLOWING DURING OR JUST AFTER THE ACTIVITY YOU DESCRIBED IN THE BOX ON THE OTHER PAGE.

1. **I felt AT EASE ...**
    ❑ 1. Not at all ❑ 2. A little ❑ 3. Moderately ❑ 4. Very much
2. **I felt AWARE, FOCUSED, and CLEAR ...**
    ❑ 1. Not at all ❑ 2. A little ❑ 3. Moderately ❑ 4. Very much
3. **My mind was CALM, QUIET, AND STILL.**
    ❑ 1. Not at all ❑ 2. A little ❑ 3. Moderately ❑ 4. Very much
4. **My hands, arms, or legs felt relaxed, WARM and HEAVY ...**
    ❑ 1. Not at all ❑ 2. A little ❑ 3. Moderately ❑ 4. Very much
5. **I was HAPPY ...**
    ❑ 1. Not at all ❑ 2. A little ❑ 3. Moderately ❑ 4. Very much
6. **I was DOZING OFF or NAPPING ...**
    ❑ 1. Not at all ❑ 2. A little ❑ 3. Moderately ❑ 4. Very much
7. **I felt THANKFUL ...**
    ❑ 1. Not at all ❑ 2. A little ❑ 3. Moderately ❑ 4. Very much
8. **I felt DISTANT and FAR AWAY from my cares and concerns ...**
    ❑ 1. Not at all ❑ 2. A little ❑ 3. Moderately ❑ 4. Very much
9. **I felt JOYFUL ...**
    ❑ 1. Not at all ❑ 2. A little ❑ 3. Moderately ❑ 4. Very much
10. **I felt "TIMELESS," "INFINITE," and "BOUNDLESS" ...**
    ❑ 1. Not at all ❑ 2. A little ❑ 3. Moderately ❑ 4. Very much
11. **My muscles felt relaxed and LIMP ...**
    ❑ 1. Not at all ❑ 2. A little ❑ 3. Moderately ❑ 4. Very much
12. **I felt LOVING ...**
    ❑ 1. Not at all ❑ 2. A little ❑ 3. Moderately ❑ 4. Very much
13. **I felt INDIFFERENT and DETACHED from my cares and concerns ...**
    ❑ 1. Not at all ❑ 2. A little ❑ 3. Moderately ❑ 4. Very much
14. **I felt AT PEACE ...**
    ❑ 1. Not at all ❑ 2. A little ❑ 3. Moderately ❑ 4. Very much
15. **My mind was SILENT AND CALM, not thinking about anything ...**
    ❑ 1. Not at all ❑ 2. A little ❑ 3. Moderately ❑ 4. Very much
16. **I felt PRAYERFUL and REVERENT ...**
    ❑ 1. Not at all ❑ 2. A little ❑ 3. Moderately ❑ 4. Very much
17. **I felt DROWSY and SLEEPY ...**
    ❑ 1. Not at all ❑ 2. A little ❑ 3. Moderately ❑ 4. Very much
18. **I felt ENERGIZED, CONFIDENT, or STRENGTHENED ...**
    ❑ 1. Not at all ❑ 2. A little ❑ 3. Moderately ❑ 4. Very much

(continued)

SRRAI

PLEASE CHECK TO WHAT EXTENT YOU FELT
EACH OF THE FOLLOWING DURING OR JUST AFTER
THE ACTIVITY YOU DESCRIBED IN THE BOX ON THE OTHER PAGE.
(continued)

19. **I felt SPIRITUAL . . .**
    ❑ 1. Not at all ❑ 2. A little ❑ 3. Moderately ❑ 4. Very much
20. **My muscles felt TIGHT, TENSE • Clenched fist or jaws • Furrowed brow**
    ❑ 1. Not at all ❑ 2. A little ❑ 3. Moderately ❑ 4. Very much
21. **I felt SAD, DEPRESSED, "BLUE"**
    ❑ 1. Not at all ❑ 2. A little ❑ 3. Moderately ❑ 4. Very much
22. **I felt PHYSICAL DISCOMFORT, PAIN • Backaches • Headaches • Fatigue**
    ❑ 1. Not at all ❑ 2. A little ❑ 3. Moderately ❑ 4. Very much
23. **I was WORRYING • Troublesome thoughts went through my mind**
    ❑ 1. Not at all ❑ 2. A little ❑ 3. Moderately ❑ 4. Very much
24. **I felt IRRITATED, ANGRY**
    ❑ 1. Not at all ❑ 2. A little ❑ 3. Moderately ❑ 4. Very much
25. **My BREATHING was NERVOUS, UNEVEN • Shallow • Hurried**
    ❑ 1. Not at all ❑ 2. A little ❑ 3. Moderately ❑ 4. Very much
26. **I felt ANXIOUS.**
    ❑ 1. Not at all ❑ 2. A little ❑ 3. Moderately ❑ 4. Very much

SRDMI

THINK BACK OVER THE PAST TWO WEEKS. TO WHAT EXTENT DID YOU EXPERIENCE THE FOLLOWING?

1. I felt AT EASE ...
❏ 1. Not at all ❏ 2. A little ❏ 3. Moderately ❏ 4. Very much
■ Would you like to feel this more ? ❏ 1. No ❏ 2. A Little ❏ 3. Somewhat more
❏ 4. Much more

2. I felt AWARE, FOCUSED, and CLEAR ...
❏ 1. Not at all ❏ 2. A little ❏ 3. Moderately ❏ 4. Very much
■ Would you like to feel this more ? ❏ 1. No ❏ 2. A Little ❏ 3. Somewhat more
❏ 4. Much more

3. My mind was CALM, QUIET AND STILL.
❏ 1. Not at all ❏ 2. A little ❏ 3. Moderately ❏ 4. Very much
■ Would you like to feel this more ? ❏ 1. No ❏ 2. A Little ❏ 3. Somewhat more
❏ 4. Much more

4. My hands, arms, or legs felt relaxed, WARM and HEAVY ...
❏ 1. Not at all ❏ 2. A little ❏ 3. Moderately ❏ 4. Very much
■ Would you like to feel this more ? ❏ 1. No ❏ 2. A Little ❏ 3. Somewhat more
❏ 4. Much more

5. I was HAPPY ...
❏ 1. Not at all ❏ 2. A little ❏ 3. Moderately ❏ 4. Very much
■ Would you like to feel this more ? ❏ 1. No ❏ 2. A Little ❏ 3. Somewhat more
❏ 4. Much more

6. I was DOZING OFF or NAPPING ...
❏ 1. Not at all ❏ 2. A little ❏ 3. Moderately ❏ 4. Very much
■ Would you like to feel this more ? ❏ 1. No ❏ 2. A Little ❏ 3. Somewhat more
❏ 4. Much more

7. I felt THANKFUL ...
❏ 1. Not at all ❏ 2. A little ❏ 3. Moderately ❏ 4. Very much
■ Would you like to feel this more ? ❏ 1. No ❏ 2. A Little ❏ 3. Somewhat more
❏ 4. Much more

8. I felt DISTANT and FAR AWAY from my cares and concerns ...
❏ 1. Not at all ❏ 2. A little ❏ 3. Moderately ❏ 4. Very much
■ Would you like to feel this more ? ❏ 1. No ❏ 2. A Little ❏ 3. Somewhat more
❏ 4. Much more

9. I felt JOYFUL ...
❏ 1. Not at all ❏ 2. A little ❏ 3. Moderately ❏ 4. Very much
■ Would you like to feel this more ? ❏ 1. No ❏ 2. A Little ❏ 3. Somewhat more
❏ 4. Much more

(continued)

SRDMI

THINK BACK OVER THE PAST TWO WEEKS. TO WHAT EXTENT DID YOU EXPERIENCE THE FOLLOWING?
(continued)

10. I felt "TIMELESS," "INFINITE," or "BOUNDLESS" ...
❏ 1. Not at all ❏ 2. A little ❏ 3. Moderately ❏ 4. Very much
■ Would you like to feel this more ? ❏ 1. No ❏ 2. A Little ❏ 3. Somewhat more
❏ 4. Much more

11. My muscles felt relaxed and LIMP ...
❏ 1. Not at all ❏ 2. A little ❏ 3. Moderately ❏ 4. Very much
■ Would you like to feel this more ? ❏ 1. No ❏ 2. A Little ❏ 3. Somewhat more
❏ 4. Much more

12. I felt LOVING ...
❏ 1. Not at all ❏ 2. A little ❏ 3. Moderately ❏ 4. Very much
■ Would you like to feel this more ? ❏ 1. No ❏ 2. A Little ❏ 3. Somewhat more
❏ 4. Much more

13. I felt INDIFFERENT and DETACHED from my cares and concerns ...
❏ 1. Not at all ❏ 2. A little ❏ 3. Moderately ❏ 4. Very much
■ Would you like to feel this more ? ❏ 1. No ❏ 2. A Little ❏ 3. Somewhat more
❏ 4. Much more

14. I felt AT PEACE ...
❏ 1. Not at all ❏ 2. A little ❏ 3. Moderately ❏ 4. Very much
■ Would you like to feel this more ? ❏ 1. No ❏ 2. A Little ❏ 3. Somewhat more
❏ 4. Much more

15. My mind was SILENT AND CALM, not thinking about anything ...
❏ 1. Not at all ❏ 2. A little ❏ 3. Moderately ❏ 4. Very much
■ Would you like to feel this more ? ❏ 1. No ❏ 2. A Little ❏ 3. Somewhat more
❏ 4. Much more

16. I felt PRAYERFUL or REVERENT ...
❏ 1. Not at all ❏ 2. A little ❏ 3. Moderately ❏ 4. Very much
■ Would you like to feel this more ? ❏ 1. No ❏ 2. A Little ❏ 3. Somewhat more
❏ 4. Much more

17. I felt DROWSY and SLEEPY ...
❏ 1. Not at all ❏ 2. A little ❏ 3. Moderately ❏ 4. Very much
■ Would you like to feel this more ? ❏ 1. No ❏ 2. A Little ❏ 3. Somewhat more
❏ 4. Much more

18. I felt ENERGIZED, CONFIDENT, or STRENGTHENED ...
❏ 1. Not at all ❏ 2. A little ❏ 3. Moderately ❏ 4. Very much
■ Would you like to feel this more ? ❏ 1. No ❏ 2. A Little ❏ 3. Somewhat more
❏ 4. Much more

SRDMI

19. I felt SPIRITUAL . . .
❏ 1. Not at all ❏ 2. A little ❏ 3. Moderately ❏ 4. Very much
■ Would you like to feel this more ? ❏ 1. No ❏ 2. A Little ❏ 3. Somewhat more
❏ 4. Much more

20. My muscles felt TIGHT, TENSE • Clenched fist or jaws • Furrowed brow
❏ 1. Not at all ❏ 2. A little ❏ 3. Moderately ❏ 4. Very much
■ Would you like to feel this less ? ❏ 1. No ❏ 2. A Little ❏ 3. Somewhat less
❏ 4. Much less

21. I felt SAD, DEPRESSED, "BLUE"
❏ 1. Not at all ❏ 2. A little ❏ 3. Moderately ❏ 4. Very much
■ Would you like to feel this less ? ❏ 1. No ❏ 2. A Little ❏ 3. Somewhat less
❏ 4. Much less

22. I felt PHYSICAL DISCOMFORT, PAIN • Backaches • Headaches • Fatigue
❏ 1. Not at all ❏ 2. A little ❏ 3. Moderately ❏ 4. Very much
■ Would you like to feel this less ? ❏ 1. No ❏ 2. A Little ❏ 3. Somewhat less
❏ 4. Much less

23. I was WORRYING • Troublesome thoughts went through my mind
❏ 1. Not at all ❏ 2. A little ❏ 3. Moderately ❏ 4. Very much
■ Would you like to feel this less ? ❏ 1. No ❏ 2. A Little ❏ 3. Somewhat less
❏ 4. Much less

24. I felt IRRITATED, ANGRY
❏ 1. Not at all ❏ 2. A little ❏ 3. Moderately ❏ 4. Very much
■ Would you like to feel this less ? ❏ 1. No ❏ 2. A Little ❏ 3. Somewhat less
❏ 4. Much less

25. My BREATHING was NERVOUS, UNEVEN • Shallow • Hurried
❏ 1. Not at all ❏ 2. A little ❏ 3. Moderately ❏ 4. Very much
■ Would you like to feel this less ? ❏ 1. No ❏ 2. A Little ❏ 3. Somewhat less
❏ 4. Much less

26. I felt ANXIOUS
❏ 1. Not at all ❏ 2. A little ❏ 3. Moderately ❏ 4. Very much
■ Would you like to feel this less ? ❏ 1. No ❏ 2. A Little ❏ 3. Somewhat less
❏ 4. Much less

SRSI

Please check to what extent you are
feeling each of the following
RIGHT NOW, AT THE PRESENT MOMENT.
Please check every statement.

1. **I feel AT EASE ...**
   ❑ 1. Not at all ❑ 2. A little ❑ 3. Moderately ❑ 4. Very Much
2. **I feel AWARE, FOCUSED, and CLEAR ...**
   ❑ 1. Not at all ❑ 2. A little ❑ 3. Moderately ❑ 4. Very Much
3. **My mind is CALM, QUIET, AND STILL.**
   ❑ 1. Not at all ❑ 2. A little ❑ 3. Moderately ❑ 4. Very Much
4. **My hands, arms, or legs feel relaxed, WARM and HEAVY ...**
   ❑ 1. Not at all ❑ 2. A little ❑ 3. Moderately ❑ 4. Very Much
5. **I am HAPPY ...**
   ❑ 1. Not at all ❑ 2. A little ❑ 3. Moderately ❑ 4. Very Much
6. **I am DOZING OFF or NAPPING ...**
   ❑ 1. Not at all ❑ 2. A little ❑ 3. Moderately ❑ 4. Very Much
7. **I feel THANKFUL ...**
   ❑ 1. Not at all ❑ 2. A little ❑ 3. Moderately ❑ 4. Very Much
8. **I feel DISTANT and FAR AWAY from my cares and concerns ...**
   ❑ 1. Not at all ❑ 2. A little ❑ 3. Moderately ❑ 4. Very Much
9. **I feel JOYFUL ...**
   ❑ 1. Not at all ❑ 2. A little ❑ 3. Moderately ❑ 4. Very Much
10. **I feel "TIMELESS," "INFINITE," or "BOUNDLESS" ...**
    ❑ 1. Not at all ❑ 2. A little ❑ 3. Moderately ❑ 4. Very Much
11. **My muscles feel relaxed and LIMP ...**
    ❑ 1. Not at all ❑ 2. A little ❑ 3. Moderately ❑ 4. Very Much
12. **I feel LOVING ...**
    ❑ 1. Not at all ❑ 2. A little ❑ 3. Moderately ❑ 4. Very Much
13. **I feel INDIFFERENT and DETACHED from my cares and concerns ...**
    ❑ 1. Not at all ❑ 2. A little ❑ 3. Moderately ❑ 4. Very Much
14. **I feel AT PEACE ...**
    ❑ 1. Not at all ❑ 2. A little ❑ 3. Moderately ❑ 4. Very Much
15. **My mind is SILENT AND CALM, not thinking about anything ...**
    ❑ 1. Not at all ❑ 2. A little ❑ 3. Moderately ❑ 4. Very Much
16. **I feel PRAYERFUL or REVERENT ...**
    ❑ 1. Not at all ❑ 2. A little ❑ 3. Moderately ❑ 4. Very Much
17. **I feel DROWSY and SLEEPY ...**
    ❑ 1. Not at all ❑ 2. A little ❑ 3. Moderately ❑ 4. Very Much
18. **I feel ENERGIZED, CONFIDENT, or STRENGTHENED ...**
    ❑ 1. Not at all ❑ 2. A little ❑ 3. Moderately ❑ 4. Very Much
19. **I feel SPIRITUAL ...**
    ❑ 1. Not at all ❑ 2. A little ❑ 3. Moderately ❑ 4. Very Much

SRSI

20. **My muscles feel TIGHT, TENSE • Clenched fist or jaws • Furrowed brow**
    ❏ 1. Not at all ❏ 2. A little ❏ 3. Moderately ❏ 4. Very Much
21. **I feel SAD, DEPRESSED, "BLUE"**
    ❏ 1. Not at all ❏ 2. A little ❏ 3. Moderately ❏ 4. Very Much
22. **I feel PHYSICAL DISCOMFORT, PAIN • Backaches • Headaches • Fatigue**
    ❏ 1. Not at all ❏ 2. A little ❏ 3. Moderately ❏ 4. Very Much
23. **I am WORRYING • Troublesome thoughts go through my mind**
    ❏ 1. Not at all ❏ 2. A little ❏ 3. Moderately ❏ 4. Very Much
24. **I feel IRRITATED, ANGRY**
    ❏ 1. Not at all ❏ 2. A little ❏ 3. Moderately ❏ 4. Very Much
25. **My BREATHING IS NERVOUS, UNEVEN • Shallow • Hurried**
    ❏ 1. Not at all ❏ 2. A little ❏ 3. Moderately ❏ 4. Very Much
26. **I feel ANXIOUS**
    ❏ 1. Not at all ❏ 2. A little ❏ 3. Moderately ❏ 4. Very Much

SRBI

WHAT DO YOU BELIEVE?
People have many beliefs and philosophies, like those below.
To what extent do you agree with each statement?
Rate each item by checking the appropriate boxes.

1. Life has a purpose greater than my personal wants and desires
    ❏ 1. Do not agree ❏ 2. Agree a little ❏ 3. Agree moderately ❏ 4. Agree very much
2. I can accept things as they are.
    ❏ 1. Do not agree ❏ 2. Agree a little ❏ 3. Agree moderately ❏ 4. Agree very much
3. God guides, loves, and comforts me.
    ❏ 1. Do not agree ❏ 2. Agree a little ❏ 3. Agree moderately ❏ 4. Agree very much
4. I believe in being direct and clear in what I say, think, and do.
    ❏ 1. Do not agree ❏ 2. Agree a little ❏ 3. Agree moderately ❏ 4. Agree very much
5. I trust the body's wisdom and healing powers.
    ❏ 1. Do not agree ❏ 2. Agree a little ❏ 3. Agree moderately ❏ 4. Agree very much
6. Sometimes it is important to simply take it easy.
    ❏ 1. Do not agree ❏ 2. Agree a little ❏ 3. Agree moderately ❏ 4. Agree very much
7. I'm optimistic about how well I will deal with my current hassles.
    ❏ 1. Do not agree ❏ 2. Agree a little ❏ 3. Agree moderately ❏ 4. Agree very much
8. It is important to love and respect others.
    ❏ 1. Do not agree ❏ 2. Agree a little ❏ 3. Agree moderately ❏ 4. Agree very much
9. There's more to life than my personal concerns and worries.
    ❏ 1. Do not agree ❏ 2. Agree a little ❏ 3. Agree moderately ❏ 4. Agree very much
10. There's no need to try to change what can't be changed.
    ❏ 1. Do not agree ❏ 2. Agree a little ❏ 3. Agree moderately ❏ 4. Agree very much
11. I put myself in God's hands.
    ❏ 1. Do not agree ❏ 2. Agree a little ❏ 3. Agree moderately ❏ 4. Agree very much
12. I believe in being honest and open with my feelings.
    ❏ 1. Do not agree ❏ 2. Agree a little ❏ 3. Agree moderately ❏ 4. Agree very much
13. There are sources of strength and healing deep within me.
    ❏ 1. Do not agree ❏ 2. Agree a little ❏ 3. Agree moderately ❏ 4. Agree very much
14. It is important to know when to stop trying, let go, and relax.
    ❏ 1. Do not agree ❏ 2. Agree a little ❏ 3. Agree moderately ❏ 4. Agree very much
15. I believe in being optimistic.
    ❏ 1. Do not agree ❏ 2. Agree a little ❏ 3. Agree moderately ❏ 4. Agree very much
16. It is important to treat people with compassion and understanding.
    ❏ 1. Do not agree ❏ 2. Agree a little ❏ 3. Agree moderately ❏ 4. Agree very much

SRCI

WHAT ARE YOUR CONCERNS?

People have many different difficulties, problems, and unmet desires. What are your concerns? In what areas are you doing OK? In what areas could you do better? Below is a list of common concerns. Please indicate the extent to which each has been a concern for you over the past two weeks. Do so by checking the appropriate box under each statement.

1. **Preparing for or recovering from surgery**
   ❑ 1. I'm doing OK ❑ 2. I could do a little better ❑ 3. I could do moderately better ❑ 4. I could do much better
2. **Artistic work**
   ❑ 1. I'm doing OK ❑ 2. I could do a little better ❑ 3. I could do moderately better ❑ 4. I could do much better
3. **Reducing my pain and discomfort**
   ❑ 1. I'm doing OK ❑ 2. I could do a little better ❑ 3. I could do moderately better ❑ 4. I could do much better
4. **Spiritual growth**
   ❑ 1. I'm doing OK ❑ 2. I could do a little better ❑ 3. I could do moderately better ❑ 4. I could do much better
5. **Managing my depression**
   ❑ 1. I'm doing OK ❑ 2. I could do a little better ❑ 3. I could do moderately better ❑ 4. I could do much better
6. **Enhancing my physical health**
   ❑ 1. I'm doing OK ❑ 2. I could do a little better ❑ 3. I could do moderately better ❑ 4. I could do much better
7. **Dealing with interpersonal conflict**
   ❑ 1. I'm doing OK ❑ 2. I could do a little better ❑ 3. I could do moderately better ❑ 4. I could do much better
8. **Enhancing my creativity**
   ❑ 1. I'm doing OK ❑ 2. I could do a little better ❑ 3. I could do moderately better ❑ 4. I could do much better
9. **Controlling my tobacco use**
   ❑ 1. I'm doing OK ❑ 2. I could do a little better ❑ 3. I could do moderately better ❑ 4. I could do much better
10. **Increasing personal strength or stamina**
    ❑ 1. I'm doing OK ❑ 2. I could do a little better ❑ 3. I could do moderately better ❑ 4. I could do much better
11. **Managing my physical symptoms**
    ❑ 1. I'm doing OK ❑ 2. I could do a little better ❑ 3. I could do moderately better ❑ 4. I could do much better
12. **Dealing with my insomnia**
    ❑ 1. I'm doing OK ❑ 2. I could do a little better ❑ 3. I could do moderately better ❑ 4. I could do much better

(continued)

SRCI

WHAT ARE YOUR CONCERNS?
(continued)

13. **Developing my ability to pray**
    ❏ 1. I'm doing OK ❏ 2. I could do a little better ❏ 3. I could do moderately better
    ❏ 4. I could do much better
14. **Managing my anxiety over medical / dental procedures**
    ❏ 1. I'm doing OK ❏ 2. I could do a little better ❏ 3. I could do moderately better
    ❏ 4. I could do much better
15. **Enhancing personal alertness and energy**
    ❏ 1. I'm doing OK ❏ 2. I could do a little better ❏ 3. I could do moderately better
    ❏ 4. I could do much better
16. **Coping with others**
    ❏ 1. I'm doing OK ❏ 2. I could do a little better ❏ 3. I could do moderately better
    ❏ 4. I could do much better
17. **Enhancing my personal insight**
    ❏ 1. I'm doing OK ❏ 2. I could do a little better ❏ 3. I could do moderately better
    ❏ 4. I could do much better
18. **Controlling my use of illegal substances**
    ❏ 1. I'm doing OK ❏ 2. I could do a little better ❏ 3. I could do moderately better
    ❏ 4. I could do much better
19. **Enhancing my sleep**
    ❏ 1. I'm doing OK ❏ 2. I could do a little better ❏ 3. I could do moderately better
    ❏ 4. I could do much better
20. **Controlling my eating problems**
    ❏ 1. I'm doing OK ❏ 2. I could do a little better ❏ 3. I could do moderately better
    ❏ 4. I could do much better
21. **Enhancing sex**
    ❏ 1. I'm doing OK ❏ 2. I could do a little better ❏ 3. I could do moderately better
    ❏ 4. I could do much better
22. **Enhancing my resistance to disease**
    ❏ 1. I'm doing OK ❏ 2. I could do a little better ❏ 3. I could do moderately better
    ❏ 4. I could do much better
23. **Preparing for or recovering from exercise workouts**
    ❏ 1. I'm doing OK ❏ 2. I could do a little better ❏ 3. I could do moderately better
    ❏ 4. I could do much better
24. **Managing the side effects of prescription medication**
    ❏ 1. I'm doing OK ❏ 2. I could do a little better ❏ 3. I could do moderately better
    ❏ 4. I could do much better
25. **Enhancing my performance at sports**
    ❏ 1. I'm doing OK ❏ 2. I could do a little better ❏ 3. I could do moderately better
    ❏ 4. I could do much better
26. **Managing my anxiety, worry, and frustration**
    ❏ 1. I'm doing OK ❏ 2. I could do a little better ❏ 3. I could do moderately better
    ❏ 4. I could do much better

SRCI

27. **Enhancing my ability to meditate**
    ❑ 1. I'm doing OK ❑ 2. I could do a little better ❑ 3. I could do moderately better
    ❑ 4. I could do much better

Index*

---

*Entries in italics indicate Relaxation Words
(R-Words)